Women's Health and Wellness

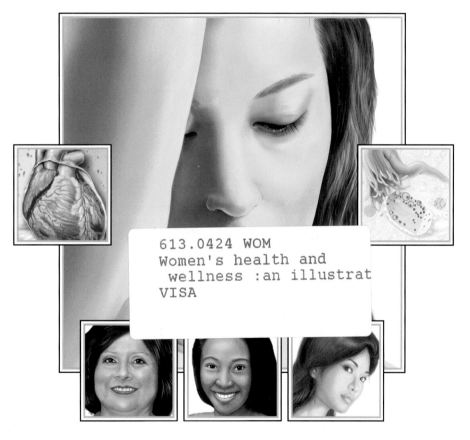

an illustrated guide

Anatomical Chart Company, Skokie, Illinois

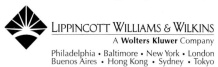

LIPPINCOTT WILLIAMS & WILKINS
A **Wolters Kluwer** Company

Philadelphia • Baltimore • New York • London
Buenos Aires • Hong Kong • Sydney • Tokyo

Published in the United States in 2002 by
ANATOMICAL CHART COMPANY
A division of Lippincott Williams & Wilkins
A Wolters Kluwer Company
8221 Kimball Avenue
Skokie, Illinois 60076-2956

This publication is not intended to be a substitute for professional medical advice,
diagnosis, or treatment. Always seek the advice of a licensed health professional with
any questions you may have regarding a medical condition. Care has been taken to
confirm the accuracy of the information. However, the publisher is not responsible
(as a matter of product liability, negligence, or otherwise) for any injury resulting
from any material contained herein.

First Edition

ISBN: 1-58779-056-4
Library of Congress Card Number: 2002103923

Developmental Editor
Lesley Weeks Ochoa

Illustrators
Dawn Gorski, M.A.M.S.
Lik Kwong, M.F.A.
Liana Bauman, M.A.M.S.

Design
Lisa Ott

Contributing Writer
Dana Demas

Medical Editor
Nancy Liskar

Production
Lisa Ott

Print and bound in the United States of America.

10 9 8 7 6 5 4 3 2 1

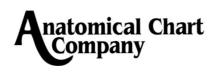

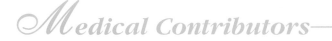

Elisabeth A. Aron, MD, FACOG
Women's Reproductive Health Scholar
University of Colorado Health Sciences Center

William E. Burkel, PhD
Professor of Anatomical Sciences
University of Michigan Medical School

Elizabeth Burns, MD, MA
Professor of Family Medicine
University of Illinois at Chicago College of Medicine

Cheryl Carmin, PhD
Associate Professor of Clinical Psychology
in Psychiatry
Director, Cognitive Behavior Therapy Program
Director, Stress and Anxiety Disorders Clinic
University of Illinois at Chicago

Seymour Diamond, MD
Director, Diamond Headache Clinic
Chicago, Illinois

David A. Fishman, MD
Professor of Obstetrics and Gynecology
Director, National Ovarian Cancer
Early Detection Program
Northwestern University
Director, Gynecologic Oncology Research
Robert H. Lurie Comprehensive Cancer Center
Northwestern University

Mark Hutchinson, MD
Associate Professor of Orthopaedics
Director of Sports Medicine Service
University of Illinois at Chicago

David A. Lipson, MD
Instructor, Pulmonary, Allergy,
and Critical Care Division
Director, Obstructive Lung Disease Program
University of Pennsylvania

Anna L. Meenan, MD, FAAFP
Assistant Professor of Family
and Community Medicine
University of Illinois College of Medicine

Laura J. Miller, MD
Associate Professor of Psychiatry
Chief of Women's Services
University of Illinois at Chicago

Ali I. Musani, MD
Interventional Pulmonologist
Hospital of the University of Pennsylvania

Jennifer O'Rourke, RN, MSN, NP
Family Nurse Practitioner
Northwestern Memorial Hospital

Bennett E. Roth, MD
Professor of Medicine
Chief of Clinical Affairs,
Division of Digestive Disease
UCLA School of Medicine

Michelle D. Seelig, MD
Family Practice Resident
University of Pennsylvania

Marla C. Solomon, RD, LD, CDE
Diabetes Educator
Evanston Northwestern Healthcare

Linda Van Horn, PhD, RD
Professor of Preventive Medicine
Research Dietitian
Northwestern University

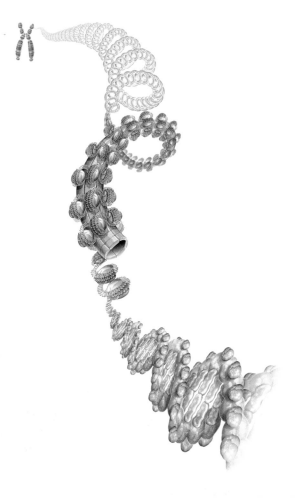

Contents

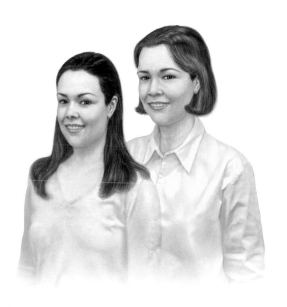

In recent years, women have been living longer and are faced with an increased incidence of cardiovascular disease, obesity, diabetes, and lung cancer. Additionally, research indicates that male and female differences go far beyond the reproductive system. It is becoming clearer that certain disease states are far more prevalent among females. As well, women's symptomatic and medication-related reactions are different than men's. Fortunately, more attention is being paid to these women's health issues.

As a female health care provider and a busy mother of three, I work both to empower my patients to be aware of their health care needs and to facilitate an ongoing dialogue of mutual respect, compassion, and friendship. Good medical knowledge, accurate references, and an empathetic practice philosophy are proven motivators for patients to take better care of themselves. Patient awareness then leads to more meaningful communication between patients and physicians.

Women today lead stressful and demanding lives and are bombarded with information, from casual conversation to the Internet. They need access to a reliable, fact-based text like *Women's Health and Wellness: An Illustrated Guide*. The book clearly illustrates the importance of caring for the female population. This text, with its start-to-finish approach, serves the information needs of women from adolescence to menopause. Designed to offer the layperson information on healthy lifestyles, disease states, nutrition, exercise, and preventive screenings by age group, it provides valuable insights and helpful suggestions.

Women's Health and Wellness is aimed at facilitating communication between patients and physicians. It serves as a quick and understandable reference guide for all women, ultimately educating readers on the uniqueness of the female body and allowing for a more proactive approach to preventive healthcare. Filled with valuable illustrations, female-specific health topics, and insights into disease processes, this book is an invaluable resource focused on integrating health behavior changes and medical management strategies. I will strongly recommend it to my patients.

Elena Kamel, M.D.
Obstetrician and Gynecologist
The Women's Group of Northwestern
Assistant Clinical Professor of Obstetrics and Gynecology
Northwestern University

*Women face a vast array of health and wellness issues over the course of a lifetime. One of the major goals of **Women's Health and Wellness: An Illustrated Guide** is to make these issues more understandable and to facilitate communication between women and their health care providers. This unique health resource uses meticulously illustrated images to teach the reader about the female body. These illustrations, along with current and concise information, make it easy to learn about women's most common health problems.*

Topics were selected for this book because of their unique application to women. All of the text is focused on women and the unique aspects of each condition as it relates to them. Topics are organized into the following sections:

- General Anatomy
- General Ailments
- Reproductive Health
- Cancers
- Healthy Aging
- Emotional Wellness
- Healthy Lifestyles

Each chapter is designed to be easy to read and visually accessible. Throughout the book, you will notice that certain words are printed in **bold** type. Definitions for these words can be found in the Glossary at the back of the book. All chapters contain quick statistical references and are organized under the following subheadings:

- Brief Definition
- Detailed Description
- Risk Factors
- Symptoms and Signs
- Prevention and Management

This book is brought to you by the Anatomical Chart Company (a subsidiary of Lippincott Williams & Wilkins) which has been providing doctors' offices with high-quality, informative medical charts for more than 30 years. The majority of the illustrations found in this guide were taken from these charts. Several leading physicians contributed their expertise to the writing of this book (please consult the credits section at the back of the book for their biographies). The information contained in Women's Health and Wellness is based on impeccable sources, such as The National Women's Health Information Center and The U.S. Department of Health and Human Services' National Institutes of Health.

We encourage women to use this guide as a springboard for more active involvement in issues of health and wellness. For more detailed information about a particular topic, please consult the On-line Sources of Information guide at the end of this book.

And remember: It is always important to seek the advice of a licensed physician for any health-related concern or question.

Enjoy!

Chapter Features

detailed description

Gives more detailed information of each topic.

DETAILED DESCRIPTION
Each month from puberty until meno
reproductive system prepares for the
An egg is released from the ovary on

risk factors

Lists the risk factors for each disorder.

RISK FACTORS
Aside from pregnancy, factors tha
periods, or heavy bleeding includ
• Hormonal fluctuations, especial

brief definition

Gives a brief description of each topic.

The menstrual cycle occurs during the reproductive period from puberty through menopause in response to rhythmic variations of hormones.

interesting facts

In the United States, the average age a girl starts menstruating is 12. However, this does not mean that all girls start at the same age. A girl can begin menstruating anytime between the ages of 8 and 16.[1]

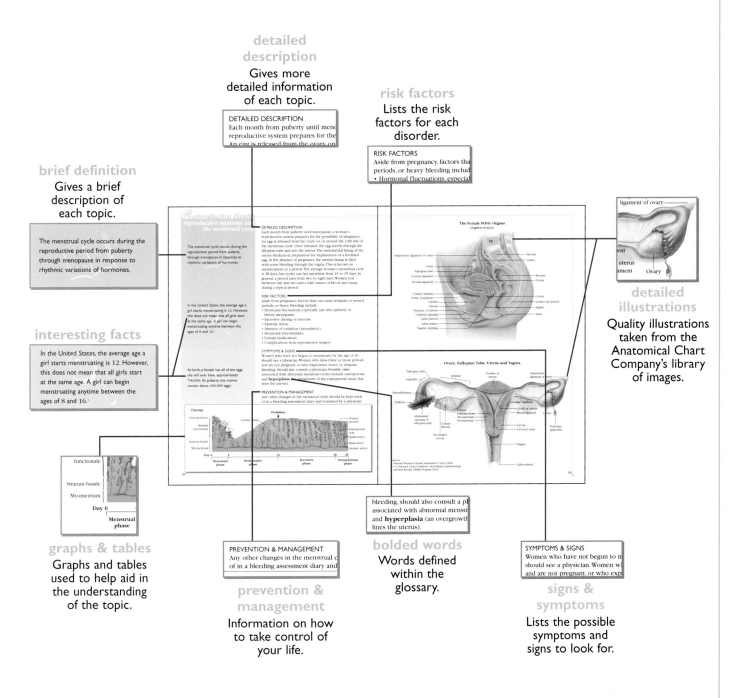

detailed illustrations

Quality illustrations taken from the Anatomical Chart Company's library of images.

graphs & tables

Graphs and tables used to help aid in the understanding of the topic.

PREVENTION & MANAGEMENT
Any other changes in the menstrual c
of in a bleeding assessment diary and

bolded words

Words defined within the glossary.

bleeding, should also consult a pl
associated with abnormal menstr
and **hyperplasia** (an overgrowth
lines the uterus).

SYMPTOMS & SIGNS
Women who have not begun to m
should see a physician. Women w
and are not pregnant, or who exp

prevention & management

Information on how to take control of your life.

signs & symptoms

Lists the possible symptoms and signs to look for.

General Anatomy

> *"Very early, I knew that the only object in life was to grow."*
> Margaret Fuller

In many ways, the skeletal, muscular, and internal organ systems of men and women are similar. However, a woman's body is distinguished from a man's by its capacity for nourishing, carrying, and giving birth to offspring. Anatomically, a woman's body goes through tremendous changes to accommodate the growth of life inside of her and to prepare for birth. A wider pelvis, a unique reproductive system, and muscles and joints that become more flexible during pregnancy—all modify the female body in a way that is completely unique and quite miraculous.

Our largest body system is called the integumentary system, which is made up of skin, hair, nails, and certain glands. This system performs many vital functions, such as protecting the muscular, skeletal, and internal organ systems.

Topics:
- Muscular System
- Skeletal System
- Internal Organs, Skin, Hair and Nail Anatomy

**Muscular System
(anterior view)**

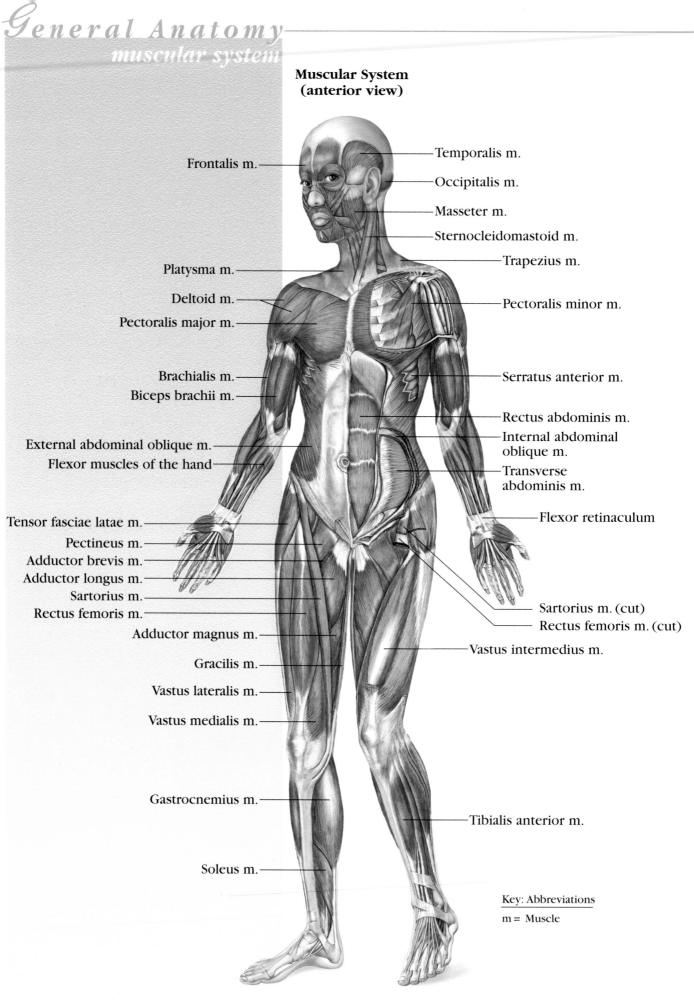

Frontalis m.

Temporalis m.

Occipitalis m.

Masseter m.

Sternocleidomastoid m.

Trapezius m.

Platysma m.

Deltoid m.

Pectoralis major m.

Pectoralis minor m.

Brachialis m.

Biceps brachii m.

Serratus anterior m.

Rectus abdominis m.

Internal abdominal
oblique m.

External abdominal oblique m.

Flexor muscles of the hand

Transverse
abdominis m.

Flexor retinaculum

Tensor fasciae latae m.

Pectineus m.

Adductor brevis m.

Adductor longus m.

Sartorius m.

Rectus femoris m.

Sartorius m. (cut)

Rectus femoris m. (cut)

Adductor magnus m.

Vastus intermedius m.

Gracilis m.

Vastus lateralis m.

Vastus medialis m.

Gastrocnemius m.

Tibialis anterior m.

Soleus m.

Key: Abbreviations

m = Muscle

Muscular System
(posterior view)

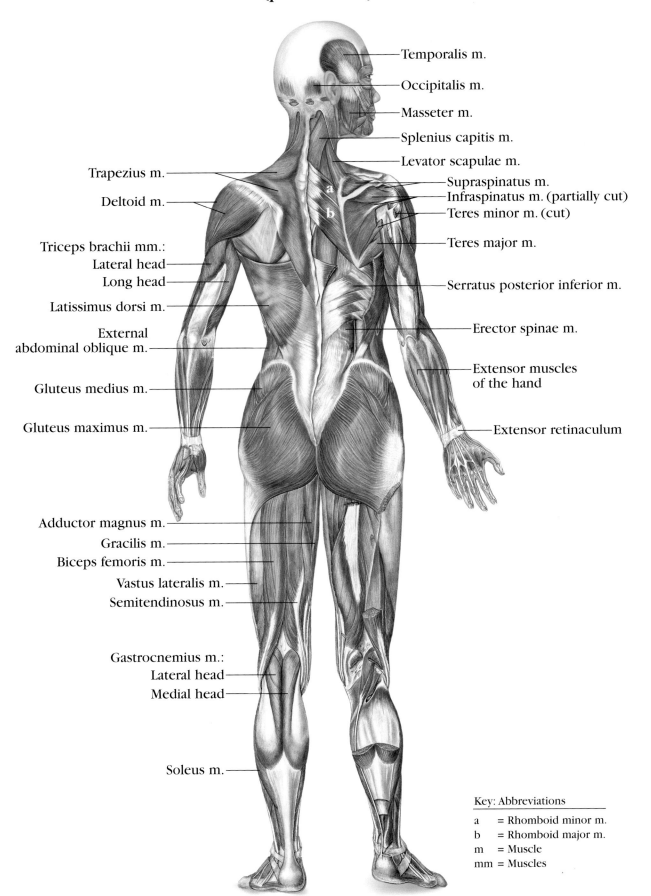

Temporalis m.

Occipitalis m.

Masseter m.

Splenius capitis m.

Levator scapulae m.

Trapezius m.

Deltoid m.

Supraspinatus m.

Infraspinatus m. (partially cut)

Teres minor m. (cut)

Teres major m.

Triceps brachii mm.:

Lateral head

Long head

Serratus posterior inferior m.

Latissimus dorsi m.

External abdominal oblique m.

Erector spinae m.

Extensor muscles of the hand

Gluteus medius m.

Gluteus maximus m.

Extensor retinaculum

Adductor magnus m.

Gracilis m.

Biceps femoris m.

Vastus lateralis m.

Semitendinosus m.

Gastrocnemius m.:

Lateral head

Medial head

Soleus m.

Key: Abbreviations

a   = Rhomboid minor m.
b   = Rhomboid major m.
m   = Muscle
mm = Muscles

4

**Skeletal System
(anterior view)**

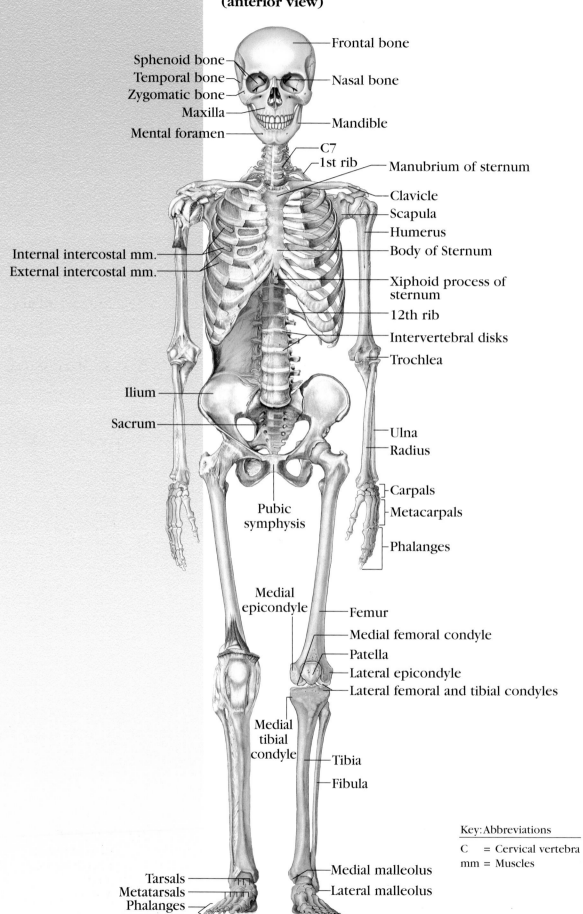

Frontal bone

Sphenoid bone

Temporal bone

Zygomatic bone

Nasal bone

Maxilla

Mental foramen

Mandible

C7

1st rib

Manubrium of sternum

Clavicle

Scapula

Humerus

Body of Sternum

Internal intercostal mm.

External intercostal mm.

Xiphoid process of
sternum

12th rib

Intervertebral disks

Trochlea

Ilium

Sacrum

Ulna

Radius

Carpals

Metacarpals

Phalanges

Pubic
symphysis

Medial
epicondyle

Femur

Medial femoral condyle

Patella

Lateral epicondyle

Lateral femoral and tibial condyles

Medial
tibial
condyle

Tibia

Fibula

Tarsals

Metatarsals

Phalanges

Medial malleolus

Lateral malleolus

Key: Abbreviations

C   = Cervical vertebra
mm = Muscles

Skeletal System
(posterior view)

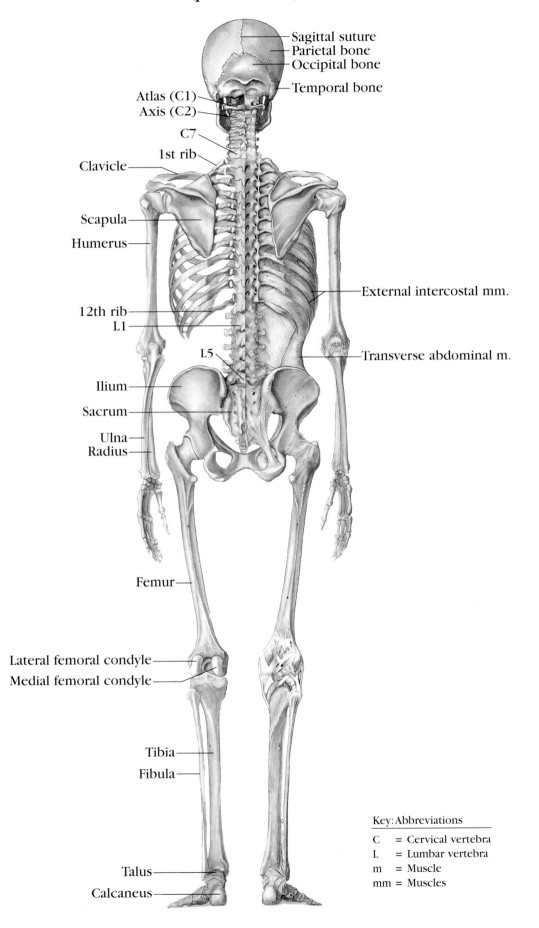

Sagittal suture
Parietal bone
Occipital bone
Temporal bone

Atlas (C1)
Axis (C2)
C7
1st rib
Clavicle
Scapula
Humerus

External intercostal mm.

12th rib
L1
L5
Ilium
Sacrum
Ulna
Radius

Transverse abdominal m.

Femur

Lateral femoral condyle
Medial femoral condyle

Tibia
Fibula

Talus
Calcaneus

Key: Abbreviations

C   = Cervical vertebra
L   = Lumbar vertebra
m   = Muscle
mm = Muscles

**Internal Organs
(anterior view)**

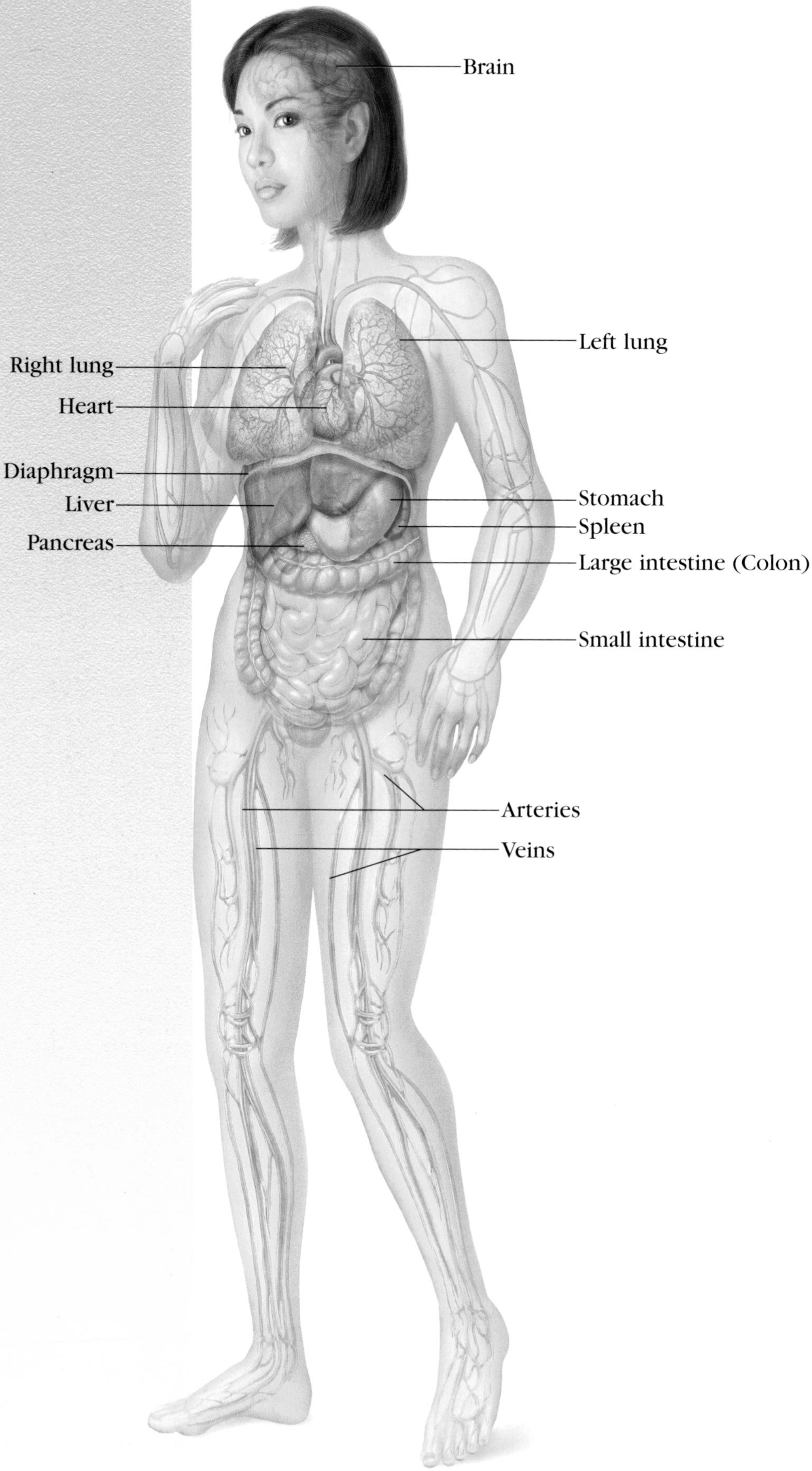

Brain

Right lung

Heart

Diaphragm

Liver

Pancreas

Left lung

Stomach

Spleen

Large intestine (Colon)

Small intestine

Arteries

Veins

The Skin

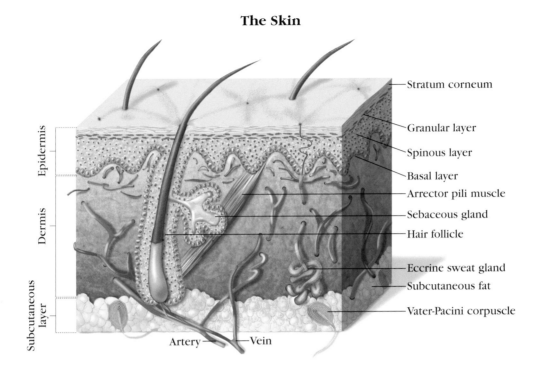

Epidermis
Dermis
Subcutaneous layer

- Stratum corneum
- Granular layer
- Spinous layer
- Basal layer
- Arrector pili muscle
- Sebaceous gland
- Hair follicle
- Eccrine sweat gland
- Subcutaneous fat
- Vater-Pacini corpuscle

Artery — Vein

Nail

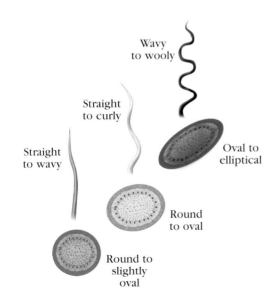

- Lateral nail fold
- Nail bed
- Nail plate
- Lunula
- Eponychium
- Nail root
- Nail matrix
- Hyponychium

Hair

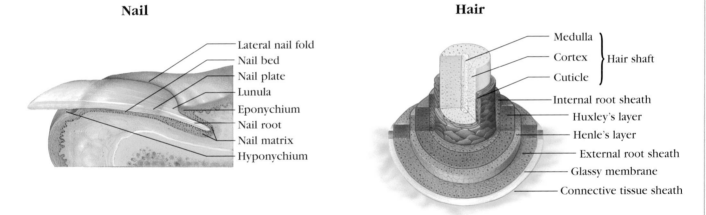

- Medulla ⎫
- Cortex ⎬ Hair shaft
- Cuticle ⎭
- Internal root sheath
- Huxley's layer
- Henle's layer
- External root sheath
- Glassy membrane
- Connective tissue sheath

Hair Fiber Characteristics

Wavy to wooly

Straight to curly

Straight to wavy

Oval to elliptical

Round to oval

Round to slightly oval

Hair-Growth Cycle

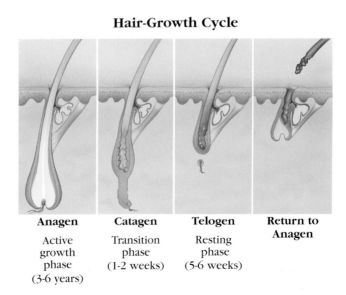

Anagen
Active growth phase
(3-6 years)

Catagen
Transition phase
(1-2 weeks)

Telogen
Resting phase
(5-6 weeks)

Return to Anagen

8

General Ailments

"Look for a long time at what pleases you, and for a longer time at what pains you."

Colette

Women experience different rates of illness, often with different symptoms, in comparison to men. For instance, women are several times more likely to develop an autoimmune disease, such as lupus or multiple sclerosis, and the symptoms of a heart attack in a woman are subtler than those a man experiences. All in all, women have unique health and wellness issues that require a different approach with the female body in mind. Good preventive care and proper management of diseases or conditions that do develop can help all women experience better health throughout their lifespan.

Topics:

Cardiovascular Disease	Allergies
Cholesterol	Lupus
Hypertension	Rheumatoid Arthritis
Heart Attack	
Stroke	Migraine Headaches
	Multiple Sclerosis
Heartburn	
Inflammatory Bowel Disease	Asthma
Irritable Bowel Syndrome	
	Incontinence
Type 1 Diabetes	Urinary Tract Infection
Type 2 Diabetes	

Cardiovascular disease includes heart disease, heart attack, and stroke.

Cardiovascular disease is the number one killer of women in America, accounting for nearly 500,000 deaths each year.[1]

More African American women die of heart disease than women of any other ethnic or racial group. Many factors could explain this, including higher rates of obesity and diabetes, and lower quality care.[2]

DETAILED DESCRIPTION

Just as the heart supplies the body's tissues and organs with blood, the heart itself needs blood to function effectively. Coronary arteries supply the heart with oxygen-rich blood. When fatty deposits narrow these arteries, a condition known as atherosclerosis occurs. Over time, narrowed arteries can become blocked, leading to heart attack, stroke and other dangerous conditions. High cholesterol, high blood pressure, and other lifestyle factors contribute significantly to the development of cardiovascular disease. Once present, these risk factors have a compounding effect on cardiovascular health. The more risk factors present, the greater the risk for developing cardiovascular disease.

RISK FACTORS

- Age.
- Family history of cardiovascular disease.
- Race.
- Smoking.
- High cholesterol.
- Hypertension (high blood pressure).
- Diabetes.
- Excess weight.
- Inadequate or lack of physical activity.

PREVENTION & MANAGEMENT

- Eat a high-fiber, low-fat, low-cholesterol diet.
- Maintain a healthy weight.
- Exercise regularly: 30 minutes of moderate physical activity on most, if not all days.
- Stop smoking, or don't start.
- Monitor cholesterol levels through regular screenings.
- Manage diabetes.

The Cardiac Cycle

Heart muscles contract (systole) and dilate (diastole) in a repeating cardiac cycle. The cycle or "heartbeat" occurs approximately 70 times per minute, pumping blood through the heart and to the body. During this cycle, deoxygenated blood enters the right side of the heart from the body and is pumped into the lungs. Oxygenated blood from the lungs enters the left side of the heart and is pumped out to the body. The illustration below demonstrates this sequence of events.

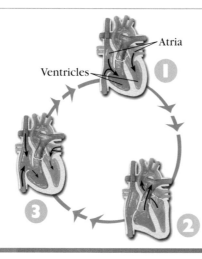

Atria

Ventricles

1 Atrial Systole
The atria contract, emptying blood into the ventricles.

2 Ventricular Systole
Shortly after atrial systole, the ventricles contract, ejecting blood from the heart to the lungs and the rest of the body.

3 Diastole
Atria and ventricles dilate and blood refills each chamber.

Anatomy of the Heart
(anterior view)

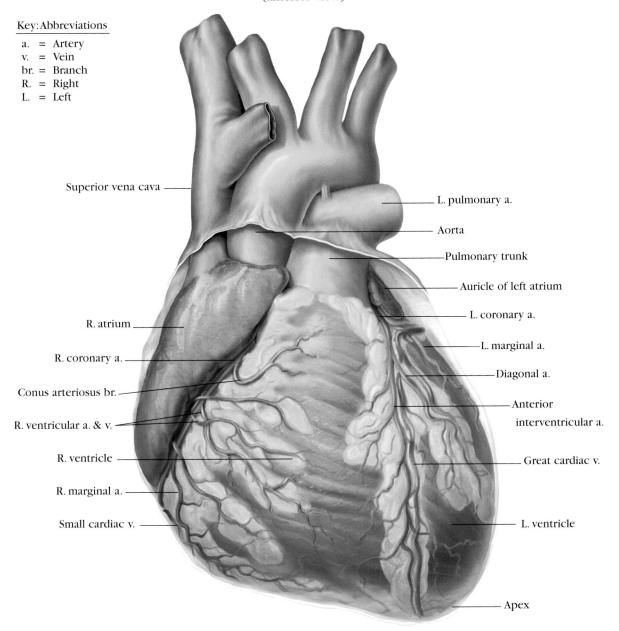

Key: Abbreviations

a. = Artery
v. = Vein
br. = Branch
R. = Right
L. = Left

Superior vena cava

L. pulmonary a.

Aorta

Pulmonary trunk

Auricle of left atrium

L. coronary a.

R. atrium

L. marginal a.

R. coronary a.

Diagonal a.

Conus arteriosus br.

Anterior interventricular a.

R. ventricular a. & v.

R. ventricle

Great cardiac v.

R. marginal a.

L. ventricle

Small cardiac v.

Apex

Progression of Cardiovascular Disease

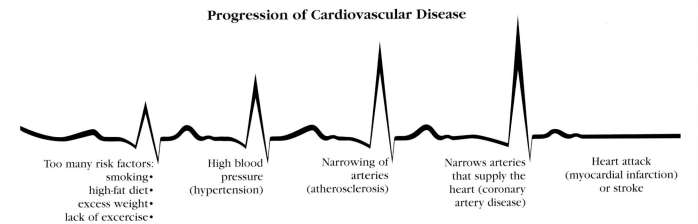

Too many risk factors: smoking• high-fat diet• excess weight• lack of excercise•

High blood pressure (hypertension)

Narrowing of arteries (atherosclerosis)

Narrows arteries that supply the heart (coronary artery disease)

Heart attack (myocardial infarction) or stroke

Sources:
1. National Women's Health Center and Centers for Disease Control, 2002.
2. National Center for Health Statistics, 2002; Agency for Healthcare
   Research and Quality, 2001.

Cholesterol is a fatty substance found naturally in your body and in high-fat foods. When the level of cholesterol in your blood becomes higher than necessary, the result is high blood cholesterol, a condition that greatly increases the risk for heart disease.

About a quarter of all American women have blood cholesterol levels high enough to pose a serious risk for heart disease. More than half of the women over age 55 need to lower their blood cholesterol.[1]

Among Hispanic women, between 43 and 52 percent have blood cholesterol above the desirable level (240mg/dL). Studies consistently indicate that dietary factors, particularly the intake of saturated fat, strongly affect the blood cholesterol levels of individuals and populations.[2]

DETAILED DESCRIPTION

Two types of cholesterol are important to heart disease. The first is low-density lipoprotein (LDL) or "bad" cholesterol, which contributes to the buildup of cholesterol in the arteries and to **atherosclerosis**. The second is high-density lipoprotein (HDL) or "good" cholesterol, which plays a protective role by helping to keep the cholesterol from building up in the arteries, thereby lowering heart disease risk. Triglycerides are another form of fat in your blood that can raise the risk of heart disease.

The HDL cholesterol level is thought to play an important role in the development of heart disease in women. A low HDL level (below 40) is strongly associated with increased heart disease risk for women.

RISK FACTORS

- Age (risk increases naturally with increasing age).
- Gender (women's LDL cholesterol levels tend to rise with menopause onset as HDL cholesterol levels decline).
- Family history of high cholesterol and/or heart disease.
- Diet high in saturated fat and cholesterol.
- Excess weight.
- Inadequate or lack of physical activity.
- Smoking.
- Diabetes.

PREVENTION & MANAGEMENT

- Eat a healthy diet that is low in saturated fat, total fat and cholesterol. Total fat should average no more than 30% of daily calories. Cholesterol should be below 300 milligrams per day.
- Exercise regularly: 30 minutes of moderate physical activity on most, if not all days.
- Maintain healthy weight.
- Stop smoking, or don't start.
- Get regular cholesterol screenings (individuals over age 20 should have cholesterol screening every 5 years or as directed by their health practitioner).
- Take prescription medications, if prescribed by the health practitioner.
- Talk to your doctor about **hormone replacement therapy (HRT)**.

Sources:
1. National Heart, Lung, and Blood Institute, 2001.
2. Office of Women's Health, 1998.
3. National Heart, Lung and Blood Institute, 2001.

For All Adults: Desired Cholesterol Levels[3]

Note: Cholesterol levels are measured in milligrams (mg) of cholesterol per deciliter (dL) of blood.

Total Cholesterol Level	Desirability
Less than 200 mg/dL	Desirable
200 – 239 mg/dL	Borderline High
240 mg/dL and above	High

LDL Cholesterol Level	Desirability
Less than 100 mg/dL	Optimal
100 - 129 mg/dL	Near Optimal/above optimal
130 – 159 mg/dL	Borderline high
160 – 189 mg/dL	High
190 mg/dL and above	Very High

HDL Cholesterol Levels
A low HDL level (less than 40) is strongly associated with increased heart disease risk for women. A level of 60 is considered protective against heart disease.

Triglycerides
Levels that are borderline high (150 –199 mg/dL) or high (200 mg/dL or more) may require treatment.

Atherosclerosis:
The Consequence of High Cholesterol

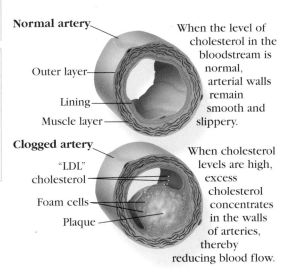

Normal artery
Outer layer
Lining
Muscle layer

When the level of cholesterol in the bloodstream is normal, arterial walls remain smooth and slippery.

Clogged artery
"LDL" cholesterol
Foam cells
Plaque

When cholesterol levels are high, excess cholesterol concentrates in the walls of arteries, thereby reducing blood flow.

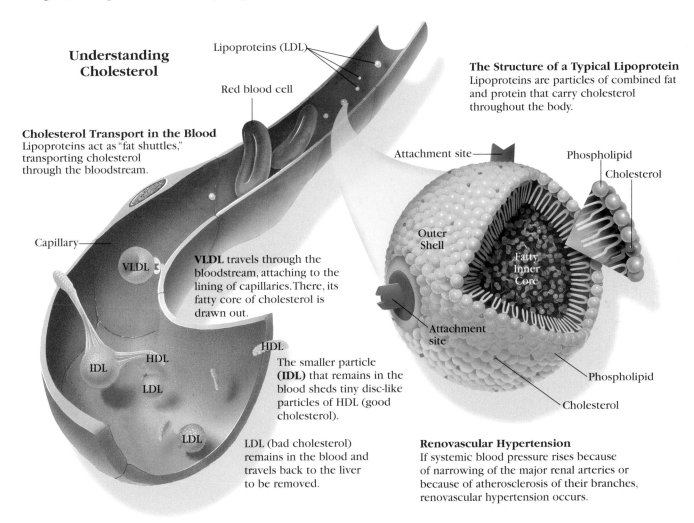

Understanding Cholesterol

Lipoproteins (LDL)

Red blood cell

Cholesterol Transport in the Blood
Lipoproteins act as "fat shuttles," transporting cholesterol through the bloodstream.

Capillary

VLDL

IDL

HDL

HDL

LDL

LDL

VLDL travels through the bloodstream, attaching to the lining of capillaries. There, its fatty core of cholesterol is drawn out.

The smaller particle **(IDL)** that remains in the blood sheds tiny disc-like particles of HDL (good cholesterol).

LDL (bad cholesterol) remains in the blood and travels back to the liver to be removed.

The Structure of a Typical Lipoprotein
Lipoproteins are particles of combined fat and protein that carry cholesterol throughout the body.

Attachment site

Phospholipid

Cholesterol

Outer Shell

Fatty Inner Core

Attachment site

Phospholipid

Cholesterol

Renovascular Hypertension
If systemic blood pressure rises because of narrowing of the major renal arteries or because of atherosclerosis of their branches, renovascular hypertension occurs.

14

Hypertension, or high blood pressure, is a disorder marked by intermittent or consistent elevation of systolic and/or diastolic blood pressure. Systolic blood pressure is measured when the heart is pumping blood out. Diastolic blood pressure is measured when the heart is resting and refilling with blood. Generally, a sustained systolic pressure of 140 mm Hg or more, or a diastolic pressure of 90 mm Hg or more, qualifies as hypertension.

African American women have high blood pressure more often than Caucasian and Hispanic women. High blood pressure affects about one-third of all African American women.[1]

More than 50 million Americans have high blood pressure, including more than half of women over the age of 60.[2]

DETAILED DESCRIPTION

Hypertension (high blood pressure) is the major cause of stroke, heart disease, and kidney failure. When blood pressure is elevated, the heart must work harder to pump blood through the arteries. Over time, this friction can lead to the development of fatty deposits in the arteries, known as atherosclerosis. In addition to the affects of atherosclorosis, stenosis (narrowing) of the major renal (kidney) arteries can contribute to **renovascular** hypertension which can also result in kidney failure.

More than half of all American women over the age of 60 suffer from high blood pressure. High blood pressure causes three of every five cases of heart failure in women.[3]

RISK FACTORS

Although the causes of high blood pressure are not entirely known, there are a number of factors that may increase a woman's risk.

- Family history of hypertension.
- Race.
- Excess weight.
- High sodium/fat diet.
- Smoking.
- Inadequate physical activity.
- Age.
- Use of oral contraceptives.
- Psychological distress.

SYMPTOMS & SIGNS

Hypertension is often referred to as the "silent killer." Many people do not realize they have hypertension until it has taken its toll on their body. In many cases, symptoms are not present and the disorder is revealed during evaluation for another disorder, or during a routine physical.

PREVENTION & MANAGEMENT

- Maintain normal body weight.
- Restrict dietary salt to no more than 2,400 milligrams a day (about 1 teaspoon).
- Eat a high-fiber, low-fat, low-cholesterol diet.
- Stop smoking, or don't start.
- Avoid excess alcohol: consume no more than one drink per day.
- Exercise regularly: 30 minutes of moderate physical activity on most, if not all days.
- Practice relaxation techniques.

Sources:
1. National Women's Health Information Center, 1999.
2. National Heart, Lung, and Blood Institute, 2002.
3. National Heart, Lung, and Blood Institute, 2002, 1998.

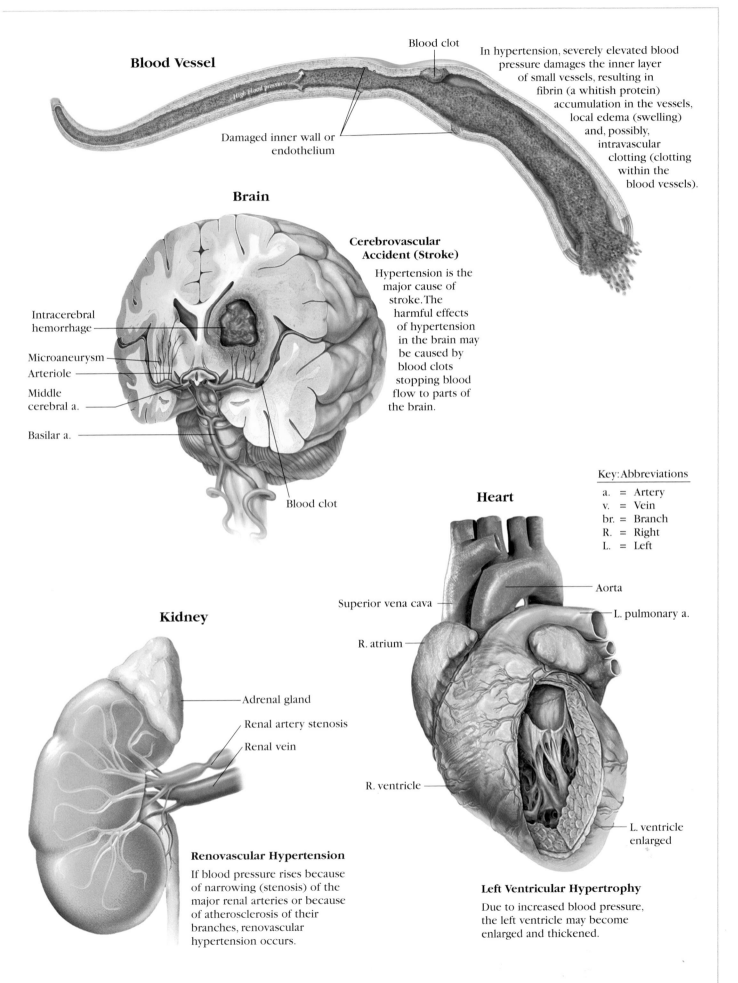

Blood Vessel

Blood clot

High blood pressure

Damaged inner wall or endothelium

In hypertension, severely elevated blood pressure damages the inner layer of small vessels, resulting in fibrin (a whitish protein) accumulation in the vessels, local edema (swelling) and, possibly, intravascular clotting (clotting within the blood vessels).

Brain

Intracerebral hemorrhage

Microaneurysm

Arteriole

Middle cerebral a.

Basilar a.

Blood clot

Cerebrovascular Accident (Stroke)

Hypertension is the major cause of stroke. The harmful effects of hypertension in the brain may be caused by blood clots stopping blood flow to parts of the brain.

Key: Abbreviations

a. = Artery
v. = Vein
br. = Branch
R. = Right
L. = Left

Heart

Aorta

Superior vena cava

L. pulmonary a.

R. atrium

R. ventricle

L. ventricle enlarged

Kidney

Adrenal gland

Renal artery stenosis

Renal vein

Renovascular Hypertension

If blood pressure rises because of narrowing (stenosis) of the major renal arteries or because of atherosclerosis of their branches, renovascular hypertension occurs.

Left Ventricular Hypertrophy

Due to increased blood pressure, the left ventricle may become enlarged and thickened.

16

A myocardial infarction, or heart attack, occurs when an area of the heart muscle dies or is damaged because of an inadequate supply of oxygen.

Each year, more than 240,000 American women suffer a heart attack. The odds of women having a second heart attack are relatively high. In fact, more women than men suffer a second heart attack within four years of their first attack.[1]

Women experience different heart attack symptoms than men do. In addition to chest pain, women are likely to have other, more subtle symptoms of heart attack.[2]

DETAILED DESCRIPTION

Myocardial infarction occurs when a coronary artery narrowed by **atherosclerosis** becomes completely blocked. This is usually the result of a blood clot that forms where the artery is narrowed. The blocked artery prevents the heart from receiving oxygen, and part or all of the heart muscle is either damaged or dies. The damaged part of the heart permanently loses its ability to contract and pump blood to and from the heart.

RISK FACTORS
- Family history of heart disease.
- Atherosclerosis.
- Hypertension.
- Smoking.
- High cholesterol.
- Diabetes.
- Obesity.
- Diet high in saturated fats.
- Inadequate physical activity.
- Use of cocaine and/or amphetamines.

SYMPTOMS & SIGNS
- Angina (chest pain).
- Neck, arm, back, or jaw discomfort.
- Shortness of breath or lightheadedness.
- Nausea.
- Sweating.
- Abdominal pain.

No two heart attacks are alike. The sooner a suspected heart attack can be treated by a medical professional, the less damage the heart will suffer.

PREVENTION & MANAGEMENT
- Maintain a normal body weight.
- Eat a high-fiber, low-fat, low-cholesterol diet.
- Stop smoking, or don't start.
- Avoid excess alcohol: consume no more than one drink per day.
- Exercise regularly: 30 minutes of moderate physical activity on most, if not all days.

Sources:
1. National Heart, Lung, and Blood Institute, 2002; National Women's Health Information Center, 2001.
2. National Heart, Lung, and Blood Institute, 2002.

Tissue Destruction in Myocardial Infarction

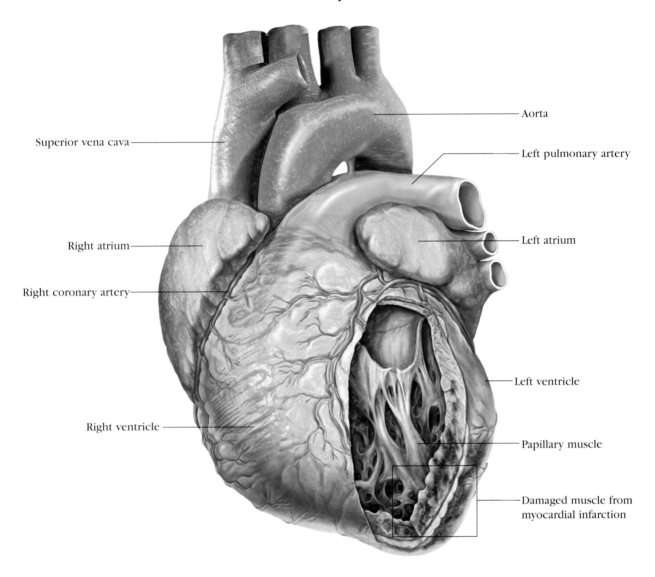

Superior vena cava

Aorta

Left pulmonary artery

Right atrium

Left atrium

Right coronary artery

Left ventricle

Right ventricle

Papillary muscle

Damaged muscle from myocardial infarction

Disease Progression of Atherosclerosis in the Blood Vessels that Leads to Myocardial Infarction

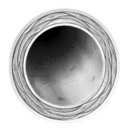

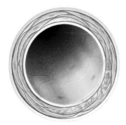

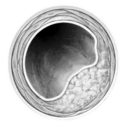

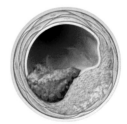

Normal

Fatty Streak

Fibrous Plaque

Calcification
with
Blood clot

The term stroke refers to the sudden death of brain tissue caused by a lack of oxygen resulting from an interruption in blood supply.

Nearly 90,000 American women die of stroke each year. As with heart attacks, women generally suffer their first stroke at a later age than men do and are more likely to die from it.[1]

Ischemic strokes are more common than hemorrhagic strokes in the United States, accounting for about 80 percent of all strokes.[2]

DETAILED DESCRIPTION

There are two main types of stroke. Ischemic strokes result from a reduction of blood flow to-or a blockage in-an artery that feeds an area of the brain. The blockage may result from **atherosclerosis** and/or blood clot formation. Hemorrhagic strokes result from bleeding within and around the brain, causing compression and tissue injury. This type of stroke can be caused by ruptured **aneurysms**, malformations in the veins or arteries, head trauma, or high blood pressure.

Many stroke victims have small strokes or warning signs before a large permanent attack. The most common are known as transient ischemic attacks (TIAs). TIAs are brief attacks that last anywhere from a few minutes to 24 hours. Many TIAs have no symptoms. Others cause temporary blindness, speaking difficulties, and/or numbness or weakness in an arm or leg.

RISK FACTORS

- Hypertension (high blood pressure).
- Family history of stroke.
- Heart disease.
- Atherosclerosis.
- Previous TIAs.
- High cholesterol.
- Obesity.
- Diabetes.
- Smoking.
- **Oral contraceptive** use, particularly in smokers over the age of 35.

SYMPTOMS & SIGNS

Although some symptoms of stroke are the same, others differ depending upon the type of stroke that occurs.

Symptoms that occur suddenly:	Ischemic	Hemmorrhagic
Weakness on one side of the body.	X	X
Numbness on one side of the body or face.	X	X
Loss of vision in one eye.	X	
Difficulty speaking or comprehending speech.	X	X
Dizziness.	X	X
Headache.	X	X
Extreme sensitivity to light.		X
Loss of consciousness.		X

Sources:
1. National Women's Health Information Center, 2002.
2. National Institute of Neurological Disorders and Stroke, 2002.

PREVENTION & MANAGEMENT

- Maintain normal blood pressure and cholesterol.
- Stop smoking or don't start.
- Eat a high-fiber, low-fat, low-cholesterol diet.
- Exercise regularly: 30 minutes of moderate physical activity on most, if not all days.
- Maintain a healthy body weight.

What Is Stroke?

The term stroke refers to the sudden death of brain tissue caused by a lack of oxygen resulting from an interrupted blood supply. An infarct is the area of the brain that has "died" because of this lack of oxygen.

Intracerebral hemorrhage

Bleeding within the brain tissue itself is known as intracerebral hemorrhage and is primarily caused by hypertension.

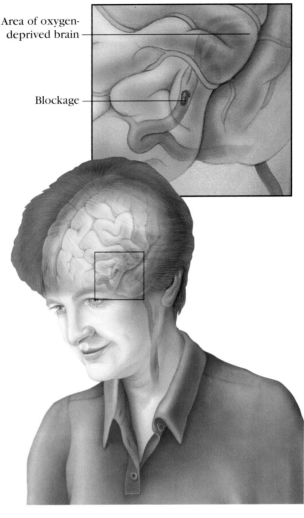

Ischemic Stroke

Area of oxygen-deprived brain

Blockage

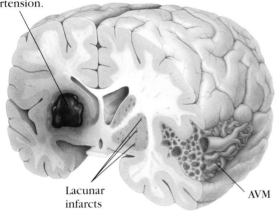

Lacunar infarcts

AVM

When a stroke occurs due to small vessel disease, a very small infarction results, sometimes called a lacunar infarction, from the French word "lacune" meaning "gap" or "cavity".

An arteriovenous malformation (AVM) is an abnormality of the brain's blood vessels in which arteries lead directly into veins without first going through a capillary bed. The pressure of the blood coming through the arteries is too high for the veins, causing them to dilate in order to transport the higher volume of blood. This dilation can cause them to rupture.

Hemorrhagic Stroke

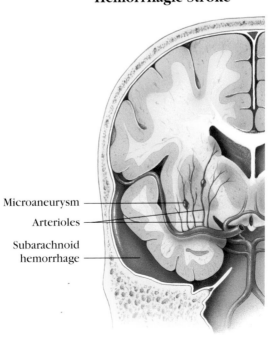

Microaneurysm

Arterioles

Subarachnoid hemorrhage

Heartburn is a burning sensation in the chest produced when acids from the stomach back up into the esophagus.

More than 60 million Americans experience heartburn at least once a month, and more than 25 million suffer heartburn symptoms every day.[1]

Twenty-five percent of pregnant women experience daily heartburn, and more than 50 percent have occasional distress.[2]

DETAILED DESCRIPTION

Heartburn is the major symptom of a condition known as gastroesophageal reflux disease (GERD). This term describes the passage of gastric, or stomach acids, up into the esophagus. Normally, a muscle between the esophagus and stomach called the lower esophageal sphincter (LES) opens temporarily to allow food into the stomach and then quickly re-closes. This mechanism prevents stomach acids from leaking into the esophagus. When the LES muscle is weakened or too relaxed, stomach acid flows backward into the esophagus. The acids irritate the lining of the esophagus. The result is the burning sensation in the chest known as heartburn.

RISK FACTORS
- Eating citrus fruits or tomatoes.
- Eating or drinking products containing peppermint or spearmint.
- Eating or drinking products containing caffeine.
- Drinking alcoholic beverages.
- Smoking.
- Obesity.
- Pregnancy.

SYMPTOMS & SIGNS
- Burning sensation in upper abdomen or chest.
- Backup of food and/or acid into throat or mouth.
- Feeling of pressure or pain in chest.
- Chronic cough.
- Recent development of asthma.
- Stomach irritation.
- Worsening of symptoms when lying down.

Heartburn that occurs once a week to once a month is considered mild to moderate. More frequent heartburn can lead to pain and can damage the lining of the esophagus, a condition called erosive esophagitis. Over time, this irritation can cause the esophagus to scar and narrow, which makes swallowing more difficult.

PREVENTION & MANAGEMENT
- Reduce consumption of irritating foods and beverages: caffeine, chocolate, alcohol, acidic fruits and vegetables (oranges, lemons, grapefruit, pineapple, tomatoes).
- Stop smoking or don't start.
- Maintain normal body weight.
- Eat smaller, more frequent meals.
- Avoid eating three hours or less before bedtime.
- When sleeping, elevate your upper torso to allow gravity to minimize the reflux of stomach acids into the esophagus.
- Take antacids.

See your doctor about diagnostic evaluation and treatment options.

Sources:
1. National Digestive Diseases Information Clearinghouse, 2001.
2. National Digestive Diseases Information Clearinghouse, 2000.

The Digestive System

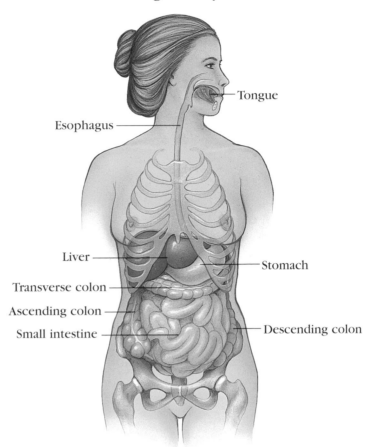

Tongue

Esophagus

Liver

Transverse colon

Ascending colon

Small intestine

Stomach

Descending colon

Normal Gastroesophageal Junction

GERD
(Gastroesophageal Reflux Disease)

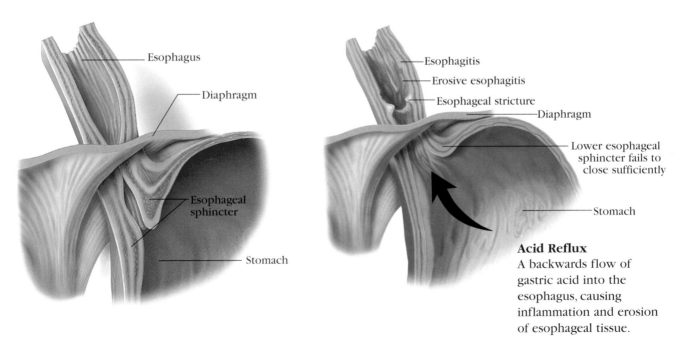

Esophagus

Diaphragm

Esophageal sphincter

Stomach

Esophagitis

Erosive esophagitis

Esophageal stricture

Diaphragm

Lower esophageal sphincter fails to close sufficiently

Stomach

Acid Reflux
A backwards flow of gastric acid into the esophagus, causing inflammation and erosion of esophageal tissue.

Inflammatory bowel disease (IBD) is a chronic condition that usually affects the intestines, rectum, and anus.

Crohn's disease and ulcerative colitis are inflammatory bowel diseases that affect nearly 2 million Americans.[1]

Patients with Crohn's disease and ulcerative colitis are at a higher risk for colorectal cancer, as compared to the general population.[2]

DETAILED DESCRIPTION

The two main types of inflammatory bowel disease (IBD) are Crohn's disease and ulcerative colitis. Crohn's disease causes inflammation in the lining and wall of the small and/or large intestine. Ulcerative colitis causes inflammation in the lining of the large intestine and rectum. In both conditions, the intestines become inflamed, which leads to **ulceration** and bleeding. IBD is usually diagnosed in people between the ages of 15 and 40. Among the 2 million Americans estimated to have IBD, equal numbers of men and women suffer from the disease.

RISK FACTORS

The causes of IBD are not known; however, about 20 percent of people with Crohn's disease have a blood relative with some form of IBD,[3] which suggests a genetic link.

SYMPTOMS & SIGNS

- Recurrent diarrhea, especially after meals.
- Abdominal pain.
- Fever.
- Constipation.
- Weight loss.
- Rectal fissure (a painful crack in the skin around the anus).
- Blood, mucus, or pus in stool.
- Red, inflamed eyes.
- Swollen joints.

In Crohn's disease, the development of fistulas (abnormal channels between the intestines and other parts of the body) can lead to the passage of stool to cavities where it should not be found, e.g. the vagina and the bladder. If food cannot be properly absorbed by the small intestine, weight loss will also occur.

PREVENTION & MANAGEMENT

Although there is no cure for IBD, it is important to seek the care of a physician early in the onset of the disease. Some people find they are able to manage their symptoms by avoiding certain foods. Most often, however, medication and nutritional supplements are used to control inflammation, correct nutritional deficiencies, and relieve symptoms. In some cases, surgery may be necessary to repair or remove damaged parts of the intestines.

Sources:
1. National Institutes of Health, Osteoporosis, and Bone Related Diseases, 1998.
2. Centers for Disease Control and Prevention, 2002.
3. National Digestive Diseases Information Clearinghouse, 2000.

Effects of Inflammatory Bowel Disease

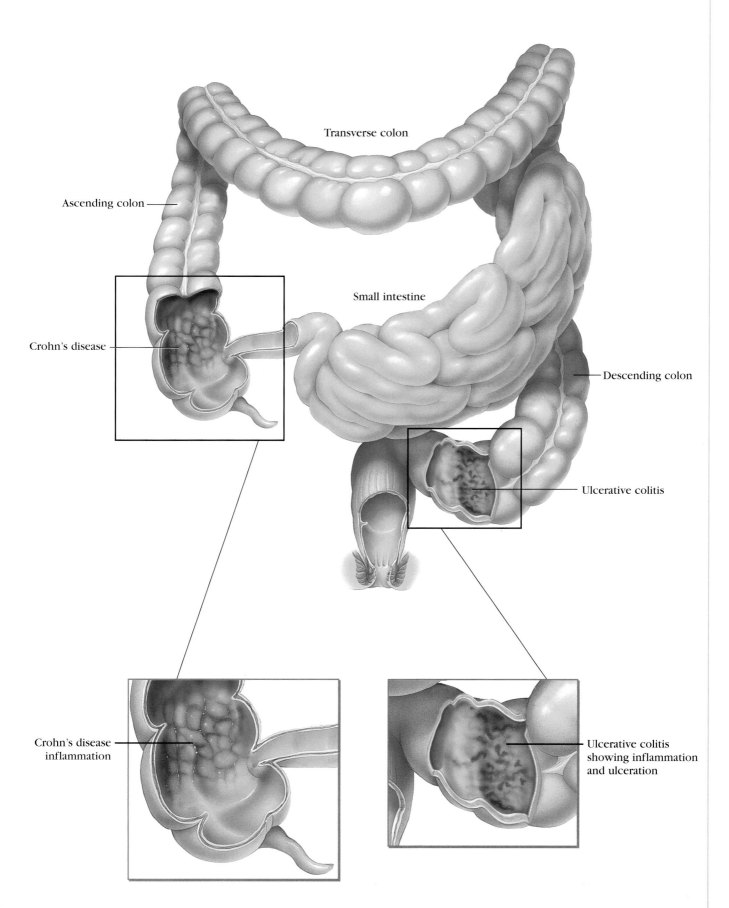

Transverse colon

Ascending colon

Small intestine

Crohn's disease

Descending colon

Ulcerative colitis

Crohn's disease inflammation

Ulcerative colitis showing inflammation and ulceration

Irritable bowel syndrome (IBS) is an intestinal disorder that causes periodic abdominal pain, bloating, and irregular bowel movements, including constipation and diarrhea.

Irritable bowel syndrome (IBS) may affect up to 20 percent of Americans–some 54 million people.[1]

The majority of people with IBS (perhaps 75 percent) are women.[2]

DETAILED DESCRIPTION

Irritable bowel syndrome (IBS) is a chronic disorder of the large intestine. Its cause is not precisely known. Doctors call it a functional disorder because there is no sign of disease when the colon is examined. The digestive tract's functioning is impaired although no tumors or inflammation within the intestines exist. The symptoms of IBS may be the result of abnormal muscle contractions within the intestines. Stress is thought to be an important trigger in IBS. IBS is typically diagnosed in late adolescence or early adulthood, almost always appearing for the first time before the age of 50.[3]

RISK FACTORS

- Stress.
- Eating high-fat foods (especially fried foods, meat, and dairy foods).
- Eating or drinking products containing caffeine.
- Drinking large amounts of alcohol.

SYMPTOMS & SIGNS

- Alternating periods of diarrhea and constipation.
- Urinary frequency and urgency.
- Painful menstruation.
- Sexual problems, such as pain during intercourse.
- Abdominal pain.
- Bloating.
- Gas.

Although the symptoms of IBS can be very uncomfortable, it does not lead to more serious intestinal problems such as cancer. It is a chronic condition that can be managed with lifestyle changes.

PREVENTION & MANAGEMENT

- Reduce consumption of irritating foods and beverages.
- Keep a food diary to determine whether certain foods make symptoms worse.
- Drink at least 6 to 8 glasses of water a day.
- Ask your physician whether a high-fiber diet is right for you.
- Practice stress management.
- Exercise regularly: 30 minutes of moderate physical activity on most, if not all days.
- Avoid alcohol.
- Eat smaller, more frequent meals and snacks.
- Take medications as prescribed by your doctor.

Sources:
1. U.S. Food and Drug Administration, 2001.
2. National Women's Health Information Center, 2002.
3. U.S. Food and Drug Administration, 2001.

Effects of Irritable Bowel Syndrome

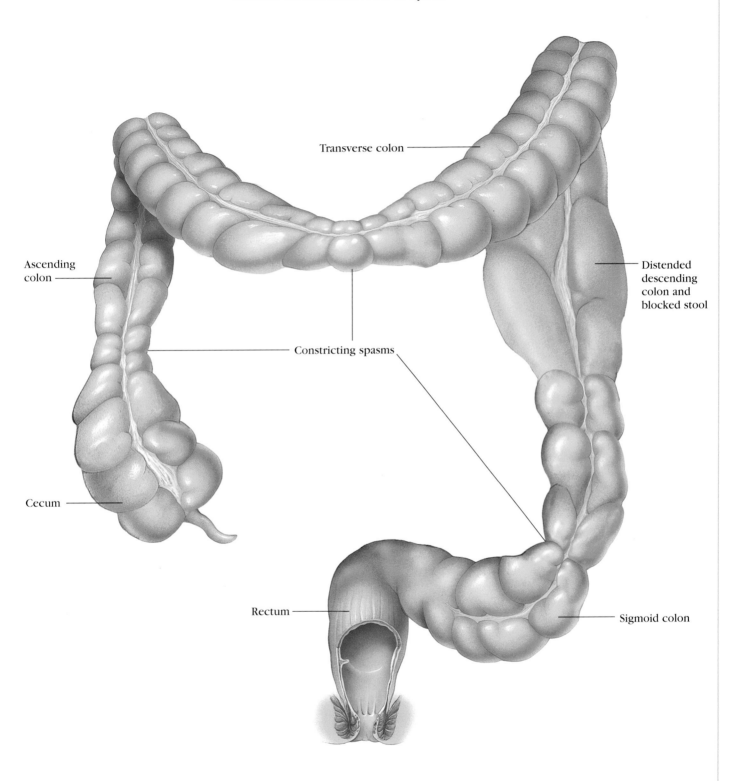

Transverse colon

Ascending colon

Distended descending colon and blocked stool

Constricting spasms

Cecum

Rectum

Sigmoid colon

Type 1 diabetes mellitus occurs when the pancreas produces little or no insulin. Insulin is needed to transport glucose from the bloodstream to the cells in order to supply energy to the body.

Type 1 diabetes affects approximately one million Americans.[1]

Type 1 diabetes occurs equally among males and females, but the disease is more common in Caucasians than non-Caucasians.[2]

DETAILED DESCRIPTION

There are two types of diabetes mellitus, Type 1 and Type 2. Most people develop Type 1 diabetes when they are children or adolescents, but it can happen at any age. Type 1 diabetes is an autoimmune disorder, which means that the body's immune system attacks its own cells (the pancreatic beta cells), which produce insulin. As a result, the pancreas produces little or no insulin. This causes glucose (blood sugar) to build up in the bloodstream, which causes complications to all body parts.

RISK FACTORS

It is unclear what causes Type 1 diabetes. A combination of genetic and environmental factors is thought to be responsible.

SYMPTOMS & SIGNS

Symptoms of Type 1 diabetes occur suddenly and may include:
• Frequent urination.
• Excessive thirst.
• Extreme hunger.
• Sudden weight loss.
• Sudden blurred vision.

PREVENTION & MANAGEMENT

There is not yet a way to prevent or cure Type 1 diabetes. With assistance from a medical diabetes team, management of the disease includes:
• Insulin medication.
• Self-monitoring of blood glucose.
• Prescribed meal plan with counting carbohydrates.
• Regular exercise.
• Regular doctor checkups.

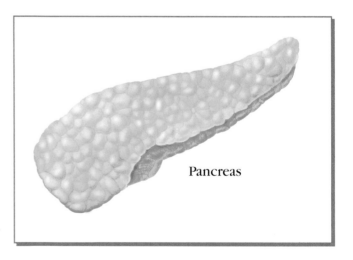

Pancreas

Sources:
1. National Institutes of Health, 2001.
2. National Diabetes Clearinghouse, 2002.

Understanding Type 1 Diabetes

2. Cellular View of Pancreas

The pancreas contains two types of secretory tissues. The exocrine portion secretes digestive juices, while the endocrine portion releases hormones. The endocrine portion consists of cells arranged in groups called the **islets of Langerhans**. The islets contain hormone-secreting cells such as alpha cells and beta cells. It is believed that the body's immune system attacks and destroys the insulin-producing beta cells.

1. Digestive System

As food enters the digestive system, it is broken down into glucose. It is either stored in the liver or absorbed into the bloodstream, where it is used by the body for energy.

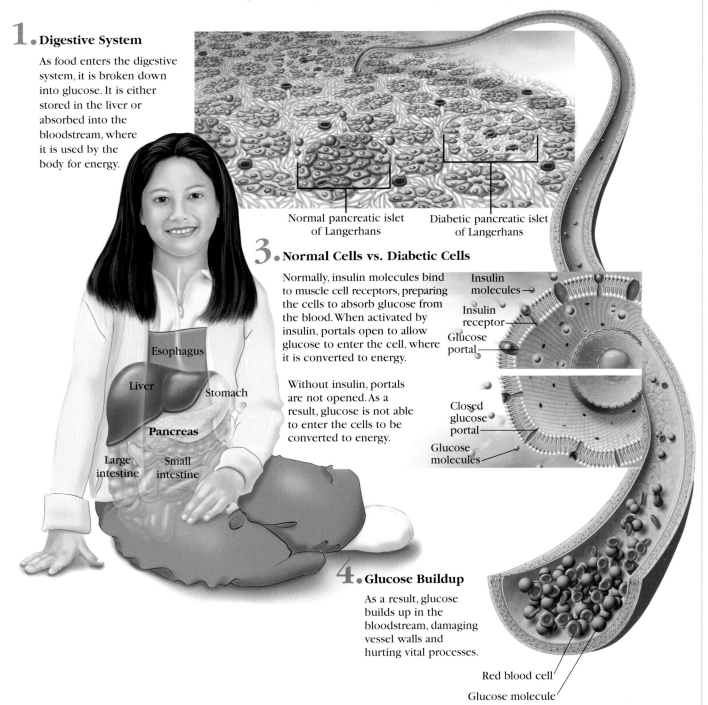

Normal pancreatic islet of Langerhans

Diabetic pancreatic islet of Langerhans

Esophagus

Liver

Stomach

Pancreas

Large intestine

Small intestine

3. Normal Cells vs. Diabetic Cells

Normally, insulin molecules bind to muscle cell receptors, preparing the cells to absorb glucose from the blood. When activated by insulin, portals open to allow glucose to enter the cell, where it is converted to energy.

Without insulin, portals are not opened. As a result, glucose is not able to enter the cells to be converted to energy.

Insulin molecules →

Insulin receptor

Glucose portal

Closed glucose portal

Glucose molecules

4. Glucose Buildup

As a result, glucose builds up in the bloodstream, damaging vessel walls and hurting vital processes.

Red blood cell

Glucose molecule

Type 2 diabetes mellitus occurs when the body's cells develop a resistance to insulin and/or when there is a decrease in insulin secretion. Insulin is needed to transport glucose from the bloodstream to the cells in order to supply energy to the body.

About 17 million people—6.2 percent of the U.S. population—have been diagnosed with Type 2 diabetes. It is estimated that another 5.9 million Americans have Type 2 diabetes but have not yet been diagnosed.[1]

Heart disease rates are three to seven times higher among women ages 45 to 64 who have diabetes than in healthy women in the same age range.[2]

DETAILED DESCRIPTION
Type 2 diabetes mellitus is the far more common type of diabetes. About 90-95 percent of women with diabetes have Type 2 diabetes.[3] It develops primarily in adults, but can also occur in children.

People with Type 2 diabetes form an insulin deficiency (lack of insulin) and/or an insulin resistance (inability to use your own insulin), which causes glucose (blood sugar) to build up in the bloodstream, causing complications in many parts of the body.

RISK FACTORS
Type 2 diabetes often develops in adults and children who are obese. Other risk factors include:
• A family history of diabetes.
• Native American, Hispanic American, or African American race or ethnicity.
• A history of diabetes during pregnancy (known as gestational diabetes).
• An inactive lifestyle.
• Age (older people are more at risk for Type 2 diabetes).
• Pre-diabetes—blood glucose levels that are higher than normal but not yet high enough to be diagnosed as diabetes.

SYMPTOMS & SIGNS
Symptoms of Type 2 diabetes may include:
• Frequent urination.
• Excessive thirst.
• Extreme hunger.
• Weight loss despite increased appetite.
• Sudden blurred vision.
• Fatigue.
• Very dry skin.
• Numbness, tingling, or pain in the legs, feet, or fingers.
• Frequent infections of the vagina, bladder, or skin.
• Sores that heal slowly.

PREVENTION & MANAGEMENT
Measures to help prevent Type 2 diabetes include:
• Maintain a healthy weight.
• Eat a high-fiber, low-fat diet.
• Exercise regularly: 30 minutes of moderate physical activity on most, if not all days.

Experts recommend that adults age 45 and older be tested for diabetes. People in high-risk groups should be tested earlier.

For people already diagnosed with Type 2 diabetes, treatment is focused on keeping the level of blood sugar (glucose) within a normal range. With assistance from a medical diabetes team, management of the disease includes:
• Meal plan to control weight, blood glucose and cholesterol.
• Blood sugar monitoring to control the disease and prevent complications.

Prevention & Management, continued.

- Diabetes medications to improve insulin release, reducing glucose and/or decrease insulin resistance.
- Exercise plan to maintain a fit body, lower blood glucose, improve cholesterol levels, and increase insulin sensitivity.
- Regular doctor checkups.

Understanding Type 2 Diabetes

Cellular View of Pancreas

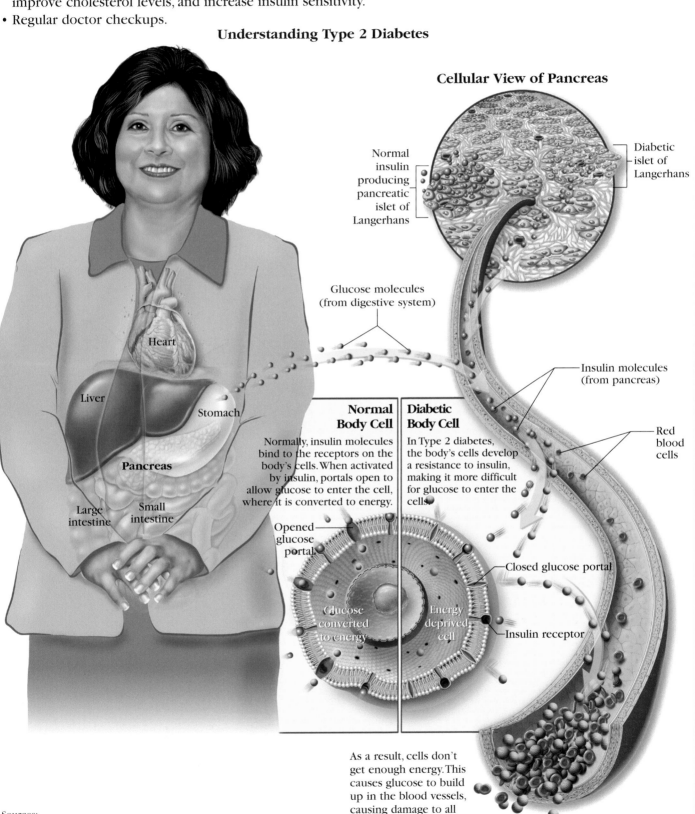

Normal insulin producing pancreatic islet of Langerhans

Diabetic islet of Langerhans

Glucose molecules (from digestive system)

Heart

Liver

Stomach

Pancreas

Large intestine

Small intestine

Insulin molecules (from pancreas)

Red blood cells

Normal Body Cell

Normally, insulin molecules bind to the receptors on the body's cells. When activated by insulin, portals open to allow glucose to enter the cell, where it is converted to energy.

Diabetic Body Cell

In Type 2 diabetes, the body's cells develop a resistance to insulin, making it more difficult for glucose to enter the cells.

Opened glucose portal

Glucose converted to energy

Energy deprived cell

Closed glucose portal

Insulin receptor

As a result, cells don't get enough energy. This causes glucose to build up in the blood vessels, causing damage to all body organs.

Sources:
1. National Diabetes Clearinghouse, 2002.
2. Centers for Disease Control and Prevention, 2001.
3. Centers for Disease Control and Prevention, 2001.

An allergy is an acquired sensitivity of the immune system. An allergic reaction occurs when the body's immune system attacks a normally harmless substance as if the substance were disease-causing. Subsequent exposures to this substance can result in physical symptoms that range from mild to life-threatening.

Allergies are the sixth leading cause of chronic disease in the United States.[1]

Approximately 16.7 million office visits to health care providers each year are attributed to allergic rhinitis, or hayfever.[2]

DETAILED DESCRIPTION

Allergens, the substances that cause allergic reactions, can enter the body in a number of different ways, including inhaling, eating/drinking, injection (as in bee venom), and contact with the skin or eyes. Common allergens include pollen, mold, animal hair or dander, dust, and certain foods (for example, peanuts, eggs, milk, wheat, and seafood). Some allergic diseases and their common symptoms include:

- Hayfever (allergic rhinitis)—sneezing, congestion, watery eyes, runny nose, along with itching of the nose, ears, or throat. A sore throat in the morning due to postnasal drip is also common.
- Allergic conjunctivitis—inflammation of the eyes associated with other allergies.
- Chronic sinusitis—inflammation of the sinuses from exposure to one or more allergens, usually lasting more than a month.
- Contact dermatitis—inflammation of the skin triggered by direct contact with an allergen.
- Eczema (atopic dermatitis)—chronic inflammation of the skin characterized by lesions, scaling, and flaking.
- Urticaria (hives)—a skin reaction with raised, reddened areas that are itchy.
- Allergic asthma—coughing, wheezing, and chest tightness after exposure to an allergen.
- Food allergy—an allergic reaction within one to two hours of ingesting a particular food. Symptoms could include swelling of lips, throat, face and tongue; upset stomach; vomiting; cramps; hives; or eczema.
- Drug allergy—a variety of allergic reactions, ranging from mild rashes to **anaphylactic shock** within minutes, that can affect any tissue or organ in the body.

RISK FACTORS

People with allergies have a genetic tendency to react to certain allergens. Exposure to those allergens may, over time, result in an allergy. Other allergic reactions, such as poison ivy contact dermatitis, are based strictly on exposures.

PREVENTION & MANAGEMENT

It is important to treat and manage the symptoms of an allergy in a timely manner. Options for treatment and prevention include:
- **Antihistamines**.
- **Corticosteroids**.
- **Immunotherapy**.
- Avoidance of the offending allergen whenever possible.

Sources:
1. American Academy of Allergy, Asthma, and Immunology, 2001.
2. Centers for Disease Control, 1999.

Respiratory Allergies

Allergies of the respiratory system are the most common types of allergies. This may be due to the large number of immune cells located along the respiratory tract and to the many potential allergens inhaled everyday. The most common inhaled allergens are from pollen, molds, dust mites, and pet dander. Hay fever and asthma are types of respiratory allergies.

Hay fever, or allergic rhinitis, is a common allergy. It is usually associated with the pollen season. The immune cells lining the nose, sinuses, eyelids and airways are very sensitive to airborne allergens, such as pollen from ragweed. Symptoms of hay fever include runny nose, sneezing, watery eyes and itchy throat. These symptoms usually occur every year at about the same time and last at least as long as the pollen is produced.

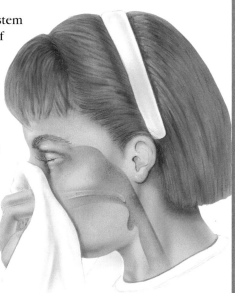

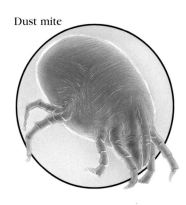

Dust mite

Household Allergies

Dust mites are microscopic organisms that live on skin tissue that is shed off regularly. The mites are commonly found on pillows, mattresses, upholstered furniture, and in clothes-changing areas. These organisms are responsible for most of the year-round type of allergic rhinitis or "hay fever."

Pathway of an Allergic Reaction

Two phases exists in allergic reactions, primary exposure and re-exposure.
In this example, the primary exposure is from allergens in the venom of an insect sting.

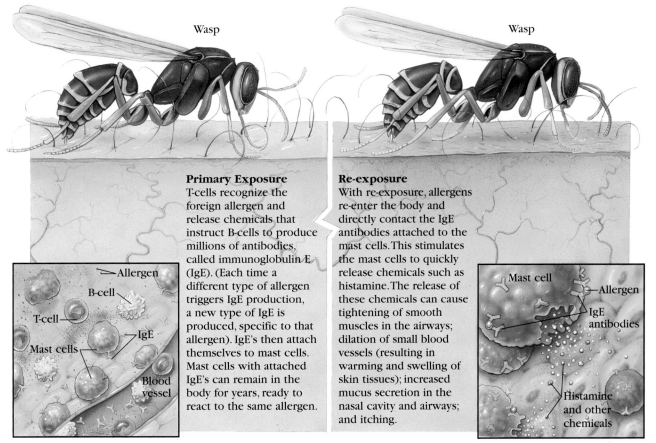

Wasp

Wasp

Primary Exposure
T-cells recognize the foreign allergen and release chemicals that instruct B-cells to produce millions of antibodies, called immunoglobulin E (IgE). (Each time a different type of allergen triggers IgE production, a new type of IgE is produced, specific to that allergen). IgE's then attach themselves to mast cells. Mast cells with attached IgE's can remain in the body for years, ready to react to the same allergen.

Re-exposure
With re-exposure, allergens re-enter the body and directly contact the IgE antibodies attached to the mast cells. This stimulates the mast cells to quickly release chemicals such as histamine. The release of these chemicals can cause tightening of smooth muscles in the airways; dilation of small blood vessels (resulting in warming and swelling of skin tissues); increased mucus secretion in the nasal cavity and airways; and itching.

Allergen
B-cell
T-cell
IgE
Mast cells
Blood vessel

Mast cell
Allergen
IgE antibodies
Histamine and other chemicals

Systemic lupus erythematosus, or lupus, is a disease that affects the body's connective tissues.

Lupus affects 1.4 million people in the United States, or 1 in every 85 people. Ninety percent of lupus patients are women.[1]

Lupus is three times more common in African American women than in Caucasian women. The disease is also more common in Hispanic American, Asian American, and Native American women.[2]

DETAILED DESCRIPTION

Lupus is a chronic autoimmune disorder, meaning that the body's immune system attacks its own cells. In lupus, the immune system attacks the body's connective tissues and organs, resulting in inflammation of the joints, blood vessels, heart, lungs, brain, or kidneys. Lupus is usually diagnosed during a woman's childbearing years.

RISK FACTORS

The cause of lupus is unknown. Experts believe lupus develops when a person inherits a predisposition for the disease and then is exposed to something in the environment, such as the following:
• An infectious agent, such as a virus.
• Extreme stress.
• In rare cases, the use of drugs such as certain tranquilizers, heart medications, and antibiotics. However, in these cases, lupus symptoms usually fade when the medications are discontinued.

SYMPTOMS & SIGNS

The symptoms associated with lupus vary greatly in frequency and severity from one person to another. Lupus symptoms tend to be vague and irregular, making diagnosis difficult. In general, lupus causes swollen joints and other symptoms for a certain period of time. Then, the disorder goes into remission, causing no symptoms for a while.

Common symptoms associated with lupus include:
• Achy or swollen joints.
• Unexplained fever.
• Extreme fatigue.
• A butterfly-shaped rash on the cheeks and nose.
• Rashes on the arms, scalp, ears, or upper torso.
• Chest pain.
• Unusual loss of hair.
• Pale or purple fingers or toes from cold or stress (called Raynaud's phenomenon).
• Sensitivity to the sun.
• Mouth and vaginal sores.
• Brain abnormalities, such as seizures or memory loss.

Sources:
1. Office on Women's Health, 2000.
2. Office on Women's Health, 2000.

PREVENTION & MANAGEMENT

There is not yet a way to prevent or cure lupus. Treatment, which focuses on reducing inflammation and minimizing symptoms, may include:

• Drugs that fight malaria.
• Anti-inflammatory drugs.
• **Corticosteroids**.
• Drugs to stop the immune system from attacking the body.

Lifestyle choices that may help manage lupus include:

• Structured exercise and rest.
• A balanced, nutritious diet.
• Avoidance of direct or prolonged sun exposure.
• Good hygiene, especially of the teeth and mouth.
• Limiting exposure to potential infections.

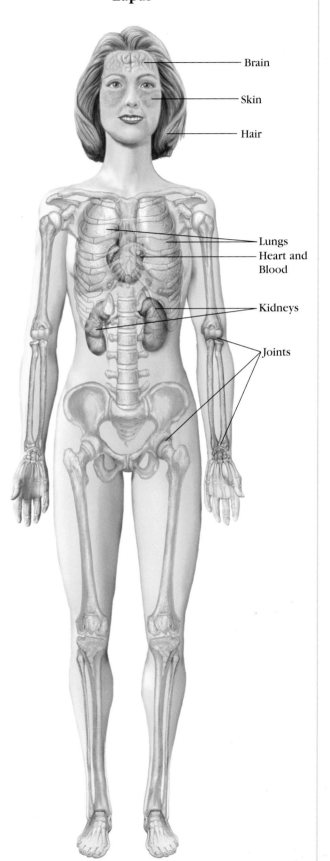

Organs Affected by Lupus

Brain

Skin

Hair

Lungs

Heart and Blood

Kidneys

Joints

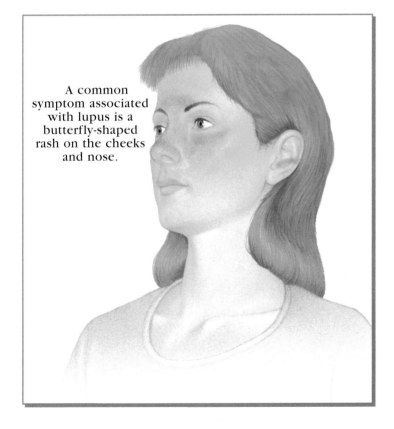

A common symptom associated with lupus is a butterfly-shaped rash on the cheeks and nose.

Rheumatoid arthritis is a chronic disease that affects the lining of the joints.

About two to three times as many women as men have rheumatoid arthritis.[1]

Scientists estimate that about 2.1 million people, or 1 percent of the U.S. adult population, have rheumatoid arthritis.[2]

DETAILED DESCRIPTION

Rheumatoid arthritis is an autoimmune disorder, meaning that the body's immune system attacks its own cells. In rheumatoid arthritis, the immune system attacks the synovium, or the smooth lining of the joints. The result is inflammation, pain, and swelling. In severe cases, rheumatoid arthritis can lead to a loss of joint function.

RISK FACTORS

The exact cause of rheumatoid arthritis is unknown. Experts think it may develop after a person who has inherited a predisposition for the disorder is exposed to a virus or some other environmental trigger.

Like all autoimmune disorders, rheumatoid arthritis is far more prevalent in women than in men. The disorder usually develops during a woman's childbearing years, between the ages of 20 and 50.

SYMPTOMS & SIGNS

The symptoms of rheumatoid arthritis vary greatly from one person to another. Common symptoms include:
• Tender, warm, and painful joints.
• A symmetrical pattern of symptoms. For example, if one knee is affected, so is the other.
• Aching or stiffness lasting for 30 minutes or longer after resting or sleeping.
• Excessive fatigue, especially in the morning.

In general, rheumatoid arthritis causes pain and other symptoms for a certain period of time. Then the disorder goes into remission, causing no symptoms for a while. Some people experience infrequent episodes and minor to moderate symptoms. But others have severe symptoms and face life-threatening complications.

PREVENTION & MANAGEMENT

There is not yet a way to prevent or cure rheumatoid arthritis. Treatment focuses on reducing inflammation and pain and slowing or stopping joint damage. Common treatment options include:
• Over-the-counter **nonsteroidal anti-inflammatory drugs (NSAIDs)**, such as aspirin, ibuprofen, and naproxen.
• **Corticosteroids**.
• Antirheumatic drugs that may slow progression of the disease.

Lifestyle choices that can help manage rheumatoid arthritis include:
• Striking a comfortable balance between rest and activity. When experiencing pain or fatigue, take a break and rest. However, too much rest may cause joint and muscle stiffness, which physical exercise can reduce.
• Heat and cold therapies to reduce the pain and inflammation of arthritis.
• Stress management and relaxation techniques.

Joints Affected by Rheumatoid Arthritis

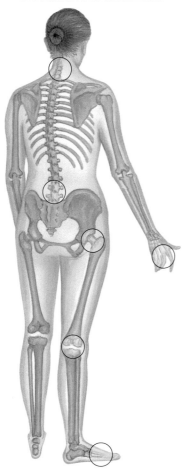

Hand and Wrist with Rheumatoid Arthritis

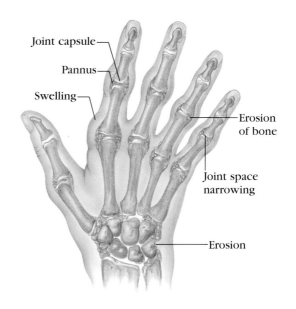

Joint capsule

Pannus

Swelling

Erosion of bone

Joint space narrowing

Erosion

Right Hip with Rheumatoid Arthritis
(anterior view)

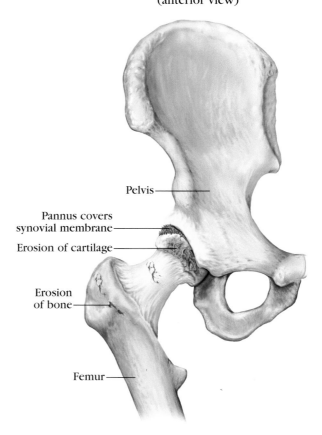

Pelvis

Pannus covers synovial membrane

Erosion of cartilage

Erosion of bone

Femur

Right Knee with Rheumatoid Arthritis
(anterior view)

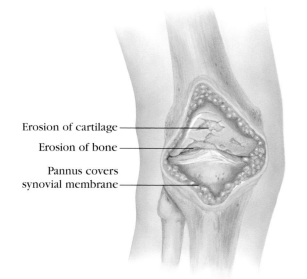

Erosion of cartilage

Erosion of bone

Pannus covers synovial membrane

Sources:
1. National Institute of Arthritis and Musculoskeletal and Skin Diseases, 1999.
2. National Institute of Arthritis and Musculoskeletal and Skin Diseases, 1999.

Headaches are a common form of pain among Americans. A migraine is a more severe, less common form of headache that involves intense, throbbing pain.

Women account for nearly 75 percent of the 28 million Americans who suffer from migraines.[1]

About 90 percent of chronic headache patients can be helped.[2]

DETAILED DESCRIPTION

A headache is a normal response to a variety of stressors, such as a cold, hunger, anxiety, or allergy. Approximately 75 percent of headaches are caused by tension in the scalp and neck muscles. A migraine headache is the second most common type of headache and accounts for approximately 18 percent of headaches experienced by women.[3]

Migraine headaches are vascular in origin. They are thought to result from changes in blood flow in the scalp and/or brain. The surface of the brain and the trigeminal nerve may be implicated in this process. When blood vessels of the head constrict, the brain is deprived of adequate oxygen. As the blood vessels respond to the lack of oxygen by widening, they release chemicals that cause pain and inflammation. The result is the intense, throbbing pain of a migraine headache.

RISK FACTORS

- Family history.
- Female gender.
- Fluctuations in hormones. Many women only experience migraines just before, during, and right after their periods. These headaches can also occur during ovulation. Most women's headaches decrease during and after menopause. However, the use of **estrogen replacement therapy (ERT)** or **oral contraceptives** may increase the frequency and severity of the attacks.

Potential triggers for migraine headaches include emotional stress, physical exertion, change in sleep patterns, bright or flickering lights, certain foods or odors, and changes in weather. Without treatment, a migraine can last anywhere from 4 to 72 hours.

SYMPTOMS & SIGNS

- Intense, throbbing pain on one or both sides of the head.
- Nausea or vomiting.
- Sensitivity to light.
- Numbness or tingling in the face.

Up to 20 percent of migraines are preceded by a group of symptoms known as an aura.[4] An aura is a group of **neurologic** symptoms that disrupt vision. Symptoms can include seeing dots, flashing lights, or dark spots.

PREVENTION & MANAGEMENT

- Monitor what triggers migraine attacks.
- Regular exercise may help some migraine sufferers. Test an exercise program to determine if it helps or aggravates the headaches.
- Practice relaxation techniques.
- Try behavioral and physical treatments, such as **acupuncture** or **biofeedback**.
- Ask your health care provider whether medication could help you.

Vascular Headaches

The Pathways of a Migraine:

A Migraine originates deep within the brain.

B Electrical impulses spread to other regions of the brain.

C Changes in nerve cell activity and blood flow may result in symptoms such as visual disturbance, numbness or tingling, and dizziness.

D Chemicals in the brain cause blood vessel dilation and inflammation of surrounding tissue.

E The inflammation irritates the trigeminal nerve, resulting in severe or throbbing pain.

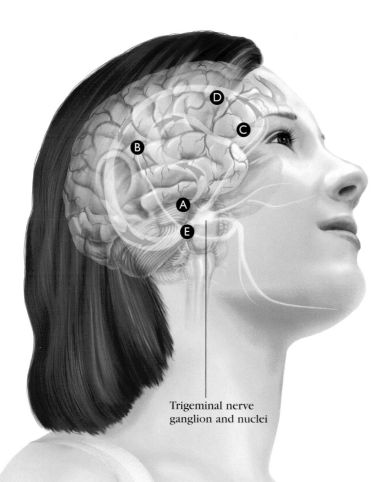

Trigeminal nerve ganglion and nuclei

I Normal blood vessel with hormone in bloodstream

Surrounding brain
Autonomic nerve
Hormone prostaglandin
Outer layer
Muscle layer
Inner layer
Lumen

II Constricted blood vessel

Surrounding brain
Autonomic nerve
Serotonin released from platelets
Red blood cells
Increase of platelets

III Dilated blood vessel

Inflammation from surrounding brain

Red blood cells
Decrease of platelets

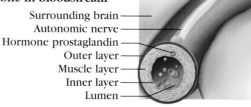

I Normal blood vessel with hormone in bloodstream

Gray matter
White matter

II Constricted blood vessel

III Dilated blood vessel

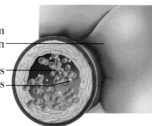

Sources:
1. National Institute of Neurological Disorders and Stroke, 2001.
2. National Institute of Neurological Disorders and Stroke, 2002.
3. American Council for Headache Education, 2000.
4. American Council for Headache Education, 2000.
Other information provided by the National Headache Foundation.

Multiple sclerosis (MS) is a progressive, debilitating disease of the central nervous system.

During her lifetime, a woman has about twice the risk of developing multiple sclerosis as a man does. Most sufferers of MS experience their first symptoms of MS between the ages of 20 and 40. Among patients who develop MS at a later age, however, the gender ratio becomes more balanced.[1]

Up to 350,000 Americans suffer from multiple sclerosis.[2]

DETAILED DESCRIPTION

Multiple sclerosis (MS) is an autoimmune disorder, meaning that the body's immune system attacks its own cells. In MS, the immune system attacks the fatty protective coating known as myelin that surrounds nerve cells in the brain and spinal cord. Myelin allows the body to transmit "messages" from one nerve cell to another. Over time, as myelin wears away, the brain's ability to transmit signals to the rest of the body is disrupted. The result is a loss of control of many bodily functions.

RISK FACTORS

The cause of MS is unknown. A person may have an increased risk of MS if there is a family history of the disease. Most people experience their first symptoms of MS between the ages of 20 and 40, but diagnosis often comes later due to the irregular nature of the disease and lack of a specific diagnostic test.

SYMPTOMS & SIGNS

People with MS experience attacks of symptoms that can last from a few days to several months. These attacks are followed by periods of remission, or symptom-free phases.
Early symptoms of MS may include:
- Feelings of tingling, burning, numbness, or pain.
- Double vision, blurry vision, or blindness.
- Unexplained weakness, dizziness, and fatigue.

During remission, the patient may feel better, but there may be lingering stiffness, weakness, numbness and vision problems. As symptoms come back, they may be more severe and include:
- Muscle spasms.
- Changes in bladder and bowel control.
- Slurred speech.
- Blindness.
- Sexual problems.
- Paralysis.
- Confusion and forgetfulness.

Most people with MS do not develop the most severe symptoms, and regain enough function to continue to lead a normal life.

PREVENTION & MANAGEMENT

There is not yet a way to prevent or cure MS. Several drugs exist that can help manage symptoms and reduce the frequency of attacks. Some non-medication treatments for managing symptoms include:
- Avoid heat: for some sufferers, heat seems to make symptoms worse.
- Practice healthy life habits to cope with fatigue and potential stress:
  - Getting enough rest.
  - Exercising regularly.
  - Eating a healthy, well-balanced diet with lots of fiber.
  - Practicing relaxation techniques.

Base of Brain

Nerve Affected by MS

Axon of
nerve

Normal
myelin
sheath

**Degenerated
myelin sheath**

Nerve fiber

**Brain Stem
and cranial nerves**

Optic nerve

Pons

Medulla oblongata

Spinal Cord

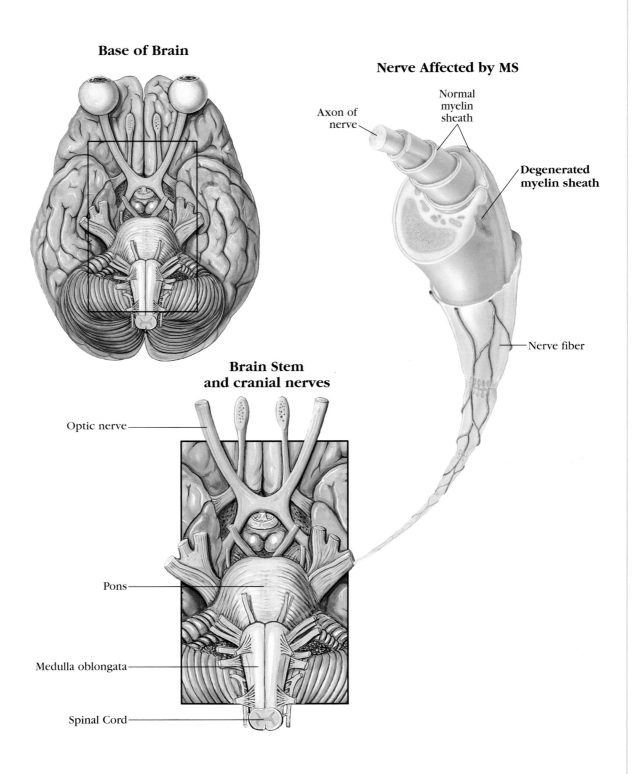

Sources:
1. National Institute of Neurological Disorders and Stroke, 2001.
2. National Institute of Neurological Disorders and Stroke, 2001.

Asthma is a chronic inflammatory disease of the lungs in which the airways become narrowed, causing such symptoms as shortness of breath, coughing, and wheezing.

In 1998, an estimated 17 million Americans, or 6.4 percent of the population, had asthma.[1]

Within the general population, asthma affects females more than males. However, among children, it affects males more.[2]

DETAILED DESCRIPTION

Asthma is a chronic condition in which the bronchial tubes of the lungs narrow, making breathing difficult. An asthma attack is the body's reaction to an irritating substance or allergen that has been inhaled. During an asthma attack, the muscles around the bronchial tubes tighten, while the lining inside the bronchial tubes becomes swollen and inflamed. Mucus production is increased, and airflow to and from the lungs becomes restricted.

RISK FACTORS

- Genetic predisposition to having overly sensitive bronchial tubes with reactive muscles.
- Presence of other allergies.
- Exposure to **aeroallergens** and irritants at less than 6 months of age.

SYMPTOMS & SIGNS

- Difficulty breathing.
- Wheezing or coughing, especially coughing at night or after exercise.
- Tightness in the neck and/or chest.

Occurrence of the above symptoms during the night is common for people suffering from uncontrolled asthma.

In a severe asthma attack, extreme shortness of breath occurs and immediate medical attention is necessary.

PREVENTION & MANAGEMENT

Asthma requires aggressive treatment involving multiple strategies to control chronic inflammation of the bronchial airways. Avoidance of allergens and a smoke-free, clean environment are essential in asthma management. Common triggers for asthma attacks include smoke, pets, plants, mold, cockroaches, house-dust mites, cold air, infection, overexertion, or extreme stress.

Asthma medications are usually taken in the form of an inhaler, although pills can be prescribed. Drugs used to treat asthma include:

- Corticosteroids—anti-inflammatory hormones that reduce inflammation and prevent future asthma attacks.
- Bronchodilators, which relax the bronchial muscles for immediate relief from asthma attacks.
- Mast cell stabilizers and leukotriene modifiers, to prevent inflammation and narrowing of the airways.

In addition, asthmatics should get yearly flu shots in order to lower the chances of having an attack.

Sources:
1. National Institute of Allergy and Infectious Diseases, 2001.
2. National Heart, Lung, and Blood Institute, Asthma Data Fact Sheet, 1999.

Respiratory System and Asthma

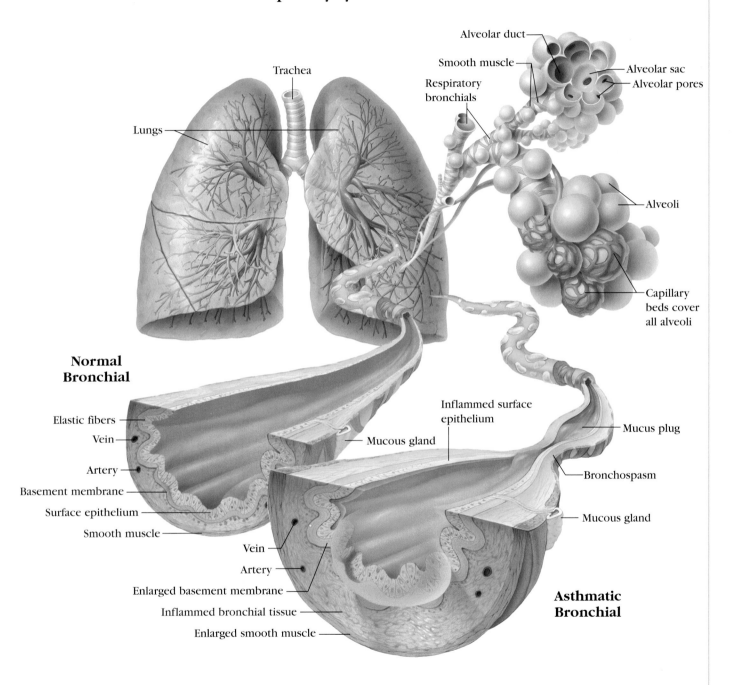

Alveolar duct

Smooth muscle

Respiratory bronchials

Alveolar sac

Alveolar pores

Trachea

Lungs

Alveoli

Capillary beds cover all alveoli

Normal Bronchial

Elastic fibers

Vein

Artery

Basement membrane

Surface epithelium

Smooth muscle

Inflammed surface epithelium

Mucous gland

Mucus plug

Bronchospasm

Mucous gland

Vein

Artery

Enlarged basement membrane

Inflammed bronchial tissue

Enlarged smooth muscle

Asthmatic Bronchial

Urinary incontinence is the involuntary loss of urine from the bladder.

As many as 13 million American women suffer from urinary incontinence. Women are two to three times more likely to experience urinary incontinence than men are.[1]

At least 1 out of 10 people age 65 or older suffers from incontinence.[2]

DETAILED DESCRIPTION

Urinary incontinence is defined as the involuntary leaking or trickling of urine from the bladder.

Stress incontinence occurs during activities that increase intra-abdominal pressure. When that pressure exceeds the pressure from the pelvic muscles that normally support the urethra, the result is involuntary urine loss. Stress incontinence is the most common form of incontinence.

Urge incontinence is characterized by an uncontrollable urge to urinate, followed by involuntary urine leakage. It is caused by spontaneous contractions of the bladder. A combination of stress and urge incontinence, called mixed incontinence, can also occur.

A less common type of incontinence, *overflow incontinence*, occurs when the pressure in a distended bladder exceeds that of the urethral pressure. This results in an almost continuous leakage of urine.

RISK FACTORS

Stress Incontinence

Since weakened pelvic muscles cause stress incontinence, a woman's risk increases if she has experienced one or more of the following:
- Pregnancy and childbirth.
- Persistent cough.
- Frequent constipation.
- Obesity.
- Menopause (lower levels of estrogen result in loss of pelvic muscle tone).

Urge Incontinence

It is not known what causes the involuntary bladder spasms that characterize urge incontinence. Risk factors associated with urge incontinence include:
- Advancing age.
- Impaired cognition (mental activities associated with thinking, learning, and memory), Alzheimer's disease.
- Parkinson's disease.
- Diabetes, stroke, multiple sclerosis.
- History of urinary tract infections.

Overflow Incontinence

Anything that causes a woman to retain urine may result in overflow incontinence. Examples are:
- Diabetes, stroke.
- Condition which causes physical immobility, such as hip fracture.
- **Pelvic prolapse.**
- Certain medications.

Sources:
1. National Kidney and Urologic Diseases Information Clearinghouse, 2000.
2. National Women's Health Information Center, 1998.

Potential triggers for incontinence include:

Trigger	Stress	Urge	Overflow
Coughing, sneezing, or laughing.	X	X	X
High-impact exercise.	X	X	
Infection.		X	
Medical conditions, such as diabetes, stroke, or multiple sclerosis.		X	X
Certain medications.		X	X

PREVENTION & MANAGEMENT
- **Kegel exercises** to strengthen the pelvic wall.
- Hormone replacement therapy (for postmenopausal women).
- **Bladder training**.
- Medication.
- Surgery.
- Management aids (absorbent pads, diapers, bedside commodes, etc.).

The Female Genitourinary System
(cross-section)

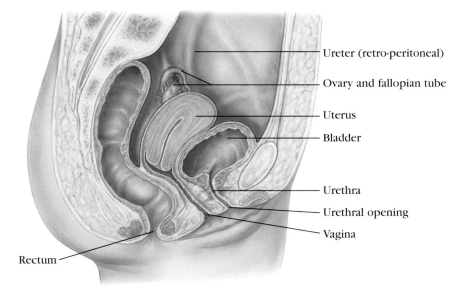

Ureter (retro-peritoneal)
Ovary and fallopian tube
Uterus
Bladder
Urethra
Urethral opening
Vagina
Rectum

The Normal Voiding Process
The voiding process, also known as micturition, is simply the steps taken by the body to expel urine from the body.

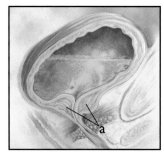

Step 1

Urine is transported from each kidney to the bladder in a long tube called the ureter. The ureters empty into the bladder which gradually fills with urine. The fluid is prevented from leaving the bladder by a thin wall of muscle at the base of the bladder. This muscle is known as the internal urethral sphincter (a). The pressure of the sphincter is greater than the pressure of the rising urine.

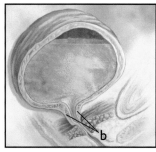

Step 2

When the bladder is full, it begins to sends messages to the brain. In turn, the brain responds with a reflex that stimulates the bladder to relax the internal urethral sphincter (b). Additionally, the main muscle of the bladder (called the detrusor muscle) begins rhythmically contracting from all sides. At the same time the urge to go to the bathroom is felt.

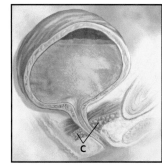

Step 3

Urine leaves the bladder by a single tube known as the urethra. When the internal sphincter relaxes, urine travels a very short distance down the first part of the urethra. However, the urine cannot leave the body while the external urethral sphincter is being clenched. When the external sphincter is relaxed (c), the urine travels down the entire urethra and leaves the body.

A urinary tract infection (UTI) occurs when bacteria enter and infect any part of the urinary tract.

Each year, 11 percent of women report suffering from at least one urinary tract infection (UTI). One in five women suffers from a UTI over the course of a lifetime.[1]

Women who have had three or more UTIs are likely to continue having them. Women with recurrent UTIs should consult their physician about preventive treatment.[2]

DETAILED DESCRIPTION

A urinary tract infection (UTI) causes inflammation and infection in the urethra, bladder, or both. In rare cases, a UTI can spread to the kidneys if left untreated. Most UTIs are caused by the E. coli bacterium, which is normally found in the intestines. Two of the ways this bacteria makes its way from the anus to a woman's urethra is during intercourse or as a result of incorrect wiping after using the bathroom. Women suffer from more UTIs than men do, in part because a woman's urethra is shorter and closer to the anus than a man's is.

RISK FACTORS

- Poor personal hygiene.
- Delaying the urge to urinate.
- Any urinary tract abnormality that obstructs the flow of urine (such as a kidney stone).
- Diabetes.

SYMPTOMS & SIGNS

- Pain or burning sensation during urination.
- Frequent urge to urinate, often without any urine produced.
- Blood in the urine.
- Pain or soreness in the lower abdomen.
- Feeling tired or shaky.
- Fever or chills.
- Low back pain.

PREVENTION & MANAGEMENT

The following can help a woman reduce her risk of developing a UTI:

- Maintain good personal hygiene.
- Wipe from front to back after using the bathroom.
- Urinate within 10 minutes after intercourse to flush out bacteria.
- Drink plenty of water.
- Drink cranberry juice to inhibit bacterial growth.
- Urinate every two to three hours during waking hours.

Most UTIs can be easily treated with antibiotics.

Sources:
1. National Kidney and Urologic Diseases Information Clearinghouse, 2001.
2. National Kidney and Urologic Diseases Information Clearinghouse, 2001.

The Female Pelvic Organs
(Sagittal section)

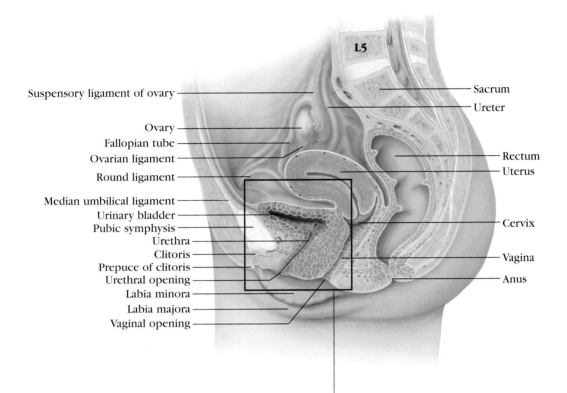

Suspensory ligament of ovary

Ovary

Fallopian tube

Ovarian ligament

Round ligament

Median umbilical ligament

Urinary bladder

Pubic symphysis

Urethra

Clitoris

Prepuce of clitoris

Urethral opening

Labia minora

Labia majora

Vaginal opening

L5

Sacrum

Ureter

Rectum

Uterus

Cervix

Vagina

Anus

Routes of Infection in the Urinary Tract

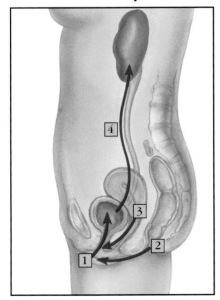

1. Ascending urethra to bladder.

2. From bowel/rectum to bladder.

3. From cervix/vagina to bladder.

4. Ascending (reflux) from bladder to kidney.

Inflammation and Infection in the Urethra and Bladder

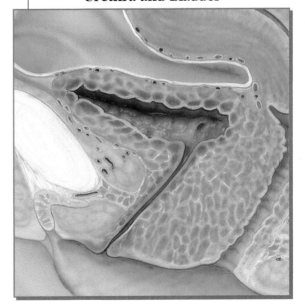

Reproductive Health

"A woman is the full circle. Within her is the power to create, nurture, and transform."

Diane Mariechild

Women are distinguished by their intricate reproductive system, located deep within the body. Over the course of a lifetime, a woman's body produces fluctuating levels of hormones, bringing about major physical changes such as the monthly menstrual cycle, pregnancy and birth, and menopause. A woman's unique biology brings with it a distinctive set of potential health concerns and benefits. Yearly Pap smears and regular visits to a gynecologist are among the best ways for women to monitor and protect their reproductive health.

Topics:
    Reproductive Anatomy and the Menstrual Cycle
    Abnormal Uterine Bleeding
    Benign Breast Lumps
    Endometriosis
    Infertility
    Pregnancy
    Labor and Birth
    Menopause: Related to Reproductive Health
    Ovarian Cysts
    Premenstrual Syndrome (PMS)
    Sexually Transmitted Disease (STDs)
    Vaginitis

The menstrual cycle occurs during the reproductive period from puberty through menopause in response to rhythmic variations of hormones.

In the United States, the average age a girl starts menstruating is 12. However, this does not mean that all girls start at the same age. A girl can begin menstruating anytime between the ages of 8 and 16.[1]

At birth, a female has all of the eggs she will ever have, approximately 700,000. At puberty, the ovaries contain about 400,000 eggs.[2]

DETAILED DESCRIPTION

Each month from puberty until menopause, a woman's reproductive system prepares for the possibility of pregnancy. An egg is released from the ovary on or around the 14th day of the menstrual cycle. Once released, the egg travels through the fallopian tube and into the uterus. The endometrial lining of the uterus thickens in preparation for implantation of a fertilized egg. In the absence of pregnancy, the uterine lining is shed with some bleeding through the vagina. This is known as menstruation, or a period. The average woman's menstrual cycle is 28 days, but cycles can last anywhere from 21 to 35 days. In general, a period lasts from two to eight days. Women lose between one and two and a half ounces of blood and tissue during a typical period.

RISK FACTORS

Aside from pregnancy, factors that can cause irregular or missed periods, or heavy bleeding include:
- Hormonal fluctuations, especially just after puberty or before menopause.
- Excessive dieting or exercise.
- Extreme stress.
- Absence of ovulation (anovulation).
- Hormonal abnormalities.
- Certain medications.
- Complications from reproductive surgery.

SYMPTOMS & SIGNS

Women who have not begun to menstruate by the age of 16 should see a physician. Women who miss three or more periods and are not pregnant, or who experience heavy or irregular bleeding, should also consult a physician. Possible risks associated with abnormal menstrual cycles include osteoporosis and hyperplasia (an overgrowth of the endometrial tissue that lines the uterus).

PREVENTION & MANAGEMENT

Any other changes in the menstrual cycle should be kept track of in a bleeding assessment diary and evaluated by a physician.

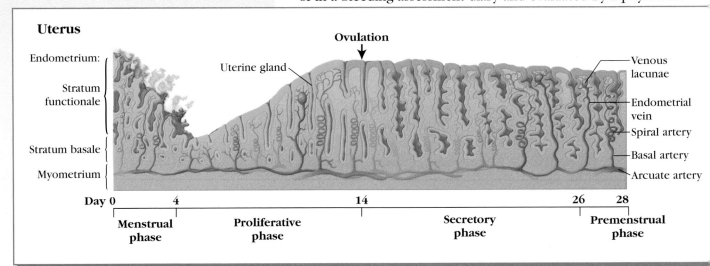

Uterus

Ovulation

Endometrium:

Stratum functionale

Uterine gland

Venous lacunae

Endometrial vein

Stratum basale

Spiral artery

Myometrium

Basal artery

Arcuate artery

Day 0   4   14   26   28

Menstrual phase | Proliferative phase | Secretory phase | Premenstrual phase

The Female Pelvic Organs
(Sagittal section)

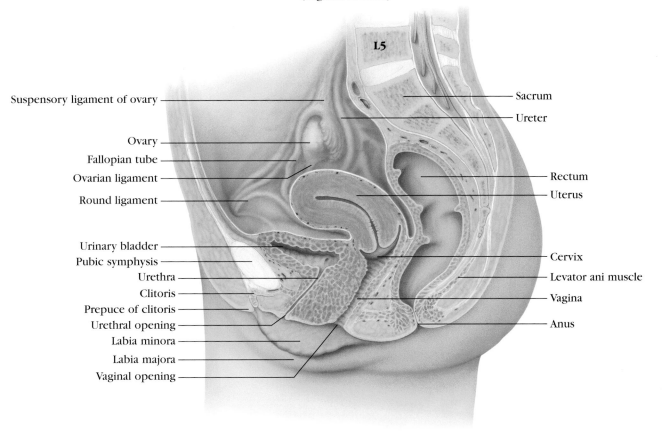

Suspensory ligament of ovary
Ovary
Fallopian tube
Ovarian ligament
Round ligament

Urinary bladder
Pubic symphysis
Urethra
Clitoris
Prepuce of clitoris
Urethral opening
Labia minora
Labia majora
Vaginal opening

L5

Sacrum
Ureter

Rectum
Uterus

Cervix
Levator ani muscle
Vagina
Anus

Ovary, Fallopian Tube, Uterus and Vagina

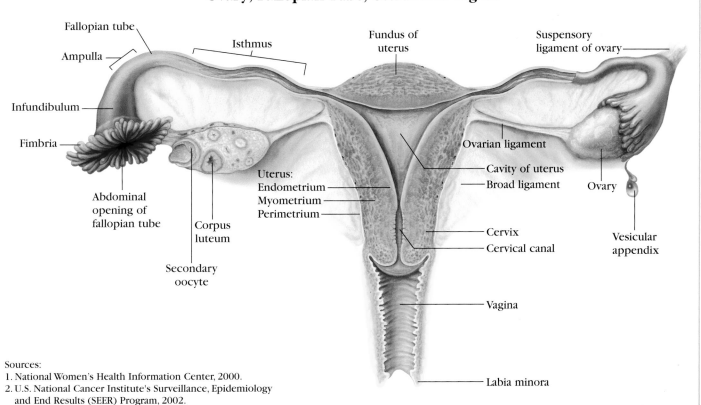

Fallopian tube
Ampulla
Infundibulum
Fimbria
Abdominal opening of fallopian tube
Corpus luteum
Secondary oocyte

Isthmus

Fundus of uterus

Uterus:
Endometrium
Myometrium
Perimetrium

Suspensory ligament of ovary

Ovarian ligament
Cavity of uterus
Broad ligament
Ovary

Cervix
Cervical canal

Vesicular appendix

Vagina

Labia minora

Sources:
1. National Women's Health Information Center, 2000.
2. U.S. National Cancer Institute's Surveillance, Epidemiology and End Results (SEER) Program, 2002.

Abnormal uterine bleeding can include excessive menstrual bleeding, bleeding at irregular times during the menstrual cycle, or the complete absence of menstrual bleeding.

It has been estimated that up to 20 to 30 percent of women of reproductive age have fibroids, though not all have been diagnosed.[1]

In the United States, 20 percent of all women of childbearing age have iron-deficiency anemia, compared with only 2 percent of adult men.[2]

DETAILED DESCRIPTION

Abnormal uterine bleeding often is the result of hormonal fluctuations or stress. Heavy or irregular uterine bleeding is common at certain times in a woman's life, such as the first few years after the start of menstruation and before menopause. In other cases, excessive or irregular bleeding may indicate a more serious problem, such as cancer. It is always important to consult your health care provider if you experience abnormal uterine bleeding.

RISK FACTORS

Common factors that cause abnormal uterine bleeding include:
- Irregular hormone production.
- Failure to **ovulate**.
- Fibroids—Non-cancerous uterine tumors that can cause excessive bleeding and/or pain.
- Cervical or endometrial polyps—small, teardrop-shaped growths on the cervix and/or lining of the uterus that are almost always non-cancerous.
- Use of certain contraceptives.
- Von Willebrand Disease—A bleeding disorder characterized by bleeding in the mucous membranes (such as the gums) and/or very heavy menstrual periods.
- **Thyroid** disorders.
- **Pituitary** disorders
- Cancer of the reproductive organs.

SYMPTOMS & SIGNS

- Heavy monthly bleeding, defined as soaking through one sanitary product every one to two hours (for several consecutive hours) or periods that last longer than seven days.
- Bleeding between periods.
- Three months without a period.
- Bleeding after menopause.
- Bleeding after intercourse.

PREVENTION & MANAGEMENT

Keep a bleeding assessment diary and consult your doctor if you notice any change in the frequency, duration, or quality of your monthly periods. Treatment may include taking iron supplements if anemia (iron deficiency) is present; in the absence of anemia, birth control pills may be prescribed. Other treatments will vary depending on the underlying condition.

Sources:
1. National Institute of Child and Human Development, 2001.
2. National Women's Health Information Center, 1998.

Common Causes of Abnormal Uterine Bleeding

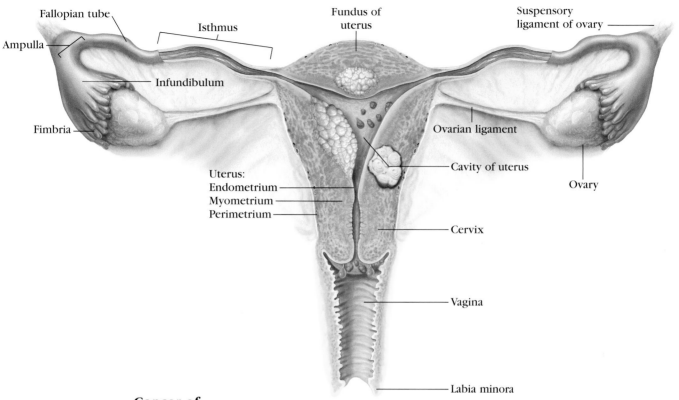

Fallopian tube

Ampulla

Isthmus

Fundus of uterus

Suspensory ligament of ovary

Infundibulum

Fimbria

Ovarian ligament

Uterus:
Endometrium
Myometrium
Perimetrium

Cavity of uterus

Ovary

Cervix

Vagina

Labia minora

Cancer of Reproductive Organs

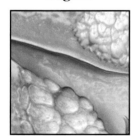

Polyps

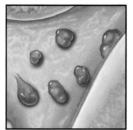

Fibroid

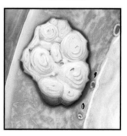

Bleeding Assessment Diary

Day of Month	Pad				Tampon				Degree of Premenstrual and Menstrual Pain
				Clots/ Flooding				Clots/ Flooding	
1									
2									
3									
4									
5									
6									

Women experience various kinds of breast lumps. Most are easily treated and some require no treatment at all.

Of breast lumps that require a biopsy, some 80 percent prove to be benign.[1]

Because they generally involve the milk-producing glandular tissues of the breast, benign breast conditions are more of a problem for women of childbearing age.[2]

DETAILED DESCRIPTION

A woman's breasts go through many changes over the course of a lifetime, as well as during each monthly menstrual cycle. Normal hormonal fluctuations are likely responsible for the growth of most benign (noncancerous) lumps in the breast.

The presence of generalized breast lumpiness is referred to as *fibrocystic changes*, *fibrocystic disease*, or *benign breast disease*. This lumpiness, which is described as "ropy" or "granular," can become more pronounced or obvious during pregnancy and as a woman approaches middle age. This condition usually requires no medical treatment.

There are several types of distinct, solitary breast lumps, the most common of which are *breast cysts* and *fibroadenomas*. Definitions of the other types of breast lumps, **fat necrosis** and **sclerosing adenosis**, can be found in the glossary.

A breast cyst is a noncancerous, fluid-filled sac that often enlarges and becomes tender just before a menstrual period. Some cysts are so small that they cannot be felt, and a very small number may grow to be several inches across. A fibroadenoma is a benign, solid, rubbery lump in the breast that can easily be moved around.

An *intraductal papilloma* is a small, noncancerous tumor that develops in the breast duct and projects into the nipple.

Though generally harmless, breast cysts, fibrodenomas, and intraductal papillomas all require some degree of medical attention and will be the focus of the majority of this chapter.

RISK FACTORS

Breast Cysts	**Fibroadenoma**	**Intraductal Papilloma**
• Age: Most common in women between the ages of 30 and 50 and tend to become less of a problem after menopause.	• Age: Most common in women in their teens and 20s, though they can occur in any age group. • Race: Occur twice as often in African American women as in other American women.	• No known risk factors. • Solitary intraductal papilloma usually affects women nearing menopause. Multiple papillomas are more common in younger women.

SYMPTOMS & SIGNS

Breast Cysts	**Fibroadenoma**	**Intraductal Papilloma**
• Detectable through breast self-examination. Cyst feels smooth and squishy if near the surface, or like a hard lump if deeper within the breast. • Cyst may grow and shrink according to monthly menstrual cycle. • Pain or discomfort in the breasts, especially around menstruation.	• Detectable through breast self-examination. Lump feels solid and rubbery. • Lump moves around the breast easily when touched and is usually painless. • Lump does not get bigger or more sensitive during monthly menstrual cycle.	• Discharge from one nipple. Can appear as clear, yellow, or bloody fluid. • Breast pain. • Breast lump. • Breast enlargement.

PREVENTION & MANAGEMENT

Although 80 percent of breast lumps are not cancerous, it is important to take steps to rule out the possibility of cancer.

• Monthly breast self-examinations.
• Annual breast exam by a trained health care provider.
• Annual mammography starting at age 40, or according to your health care provider's recommendation.
• Any breast lumps or breast changes should be checked out by a health care professional.

Treatment options vary by condition:

• Treatment for fibrocystic disease focuses on relieving the symptoms, which includes wearing a supportive bra, taking mild anti-inflammatory drugs, and regulating the menstrual cycle with the use of **oral contraceptives**.
• Breast cysts are usually treated by observation or by withdrawing fluid with a needle.
• Although fibroadenomas do not become malignant, they can enlarge with pregnancy and breast-feeding. Most surgeons believe that it is a good idea to remove fibroadenomas to make sure they are benign.
• Multiple intraductal papillomas, or any papillomas associated with a lump, need to be removed.

Normal Breast Anatomy

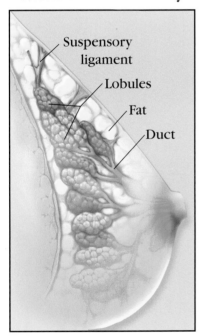

Suspensory ligament
Lobules
Fat
Duct

Fibrocystic Disease

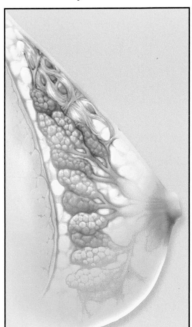

Breast Cyst

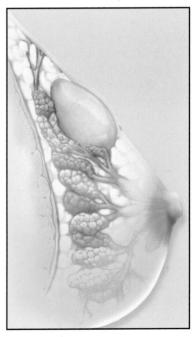

Sources:
1. National Cancer Institute, 2002.
2. National Cancer Institute, 2002.

Endometriosis occurs when the endometrium—the tissue that normally lines the uterus—grows outside the uterus and in other areas of the body.

It is estimated that between 10 and 20 percent of American women of childbearing age have endometriosis.[1]

Endometrial cancer is very rarely associated with endometriosis, occurring in less than 1 percent of women who have the disease.[2]

DETAILED DESCRIPTION

Each month, the endometrial tissue that lines the uterus normally thickens with blood in preparation for a fertilized egg. If an egg is not fertilized, the tissue is shed through menstruation. With endometriosis, however, the tissue grows outside the uterus, often on the ovaries or fallopian tubes, but sometimes in other parts of the abdomen. Since the endometrial tissue is not expelled from the body, inflammation and scarring of surrounding tissue occur. It is not known precisely what causes endometriosis, but possible causes include the reflux of menstrual blood into the fallopian tubes and coelomic metaplasia, in which a type of pelvic tissue known as coelomic epithelium is transformed into enodmetrium-like tissue. In addition, there may be an **immunologic** component to this disease.

RISK FACTORS

Although the cause is still unknown, risk factors for endometriosis include:
- Family history of endometriosis.
- Conditions associated with high levels of estrogen, such as early menstruation; longer, heavier menstrual cycles; and irregular cycles.

SYMPTOMS & SIGNS

The symptoms associated with endometriosis vary from woman to woman and can be difficult to define. In some cases, endometriosis produces no symptoms. Some of the most common symptoms include:
- Pain that follows a certain pattern during each menstrual cycle—usually increasing pain just before and during a period.
- Dyspareunia, or sharp pelvic pain during or after intercourse, especially during periods.
- Painful bowel movements during periods.
- Difficulty achieving pregnancy.
- Painful urination.
- Blood in the urine or stool.
- Lower backaches during periods.

PREVENTION & MANAGEMENT

In order to diagnose endometriosis, a doctor must perform a procedure called a **laparoscopy** to determine if endometriosis is present. Abnormal tissue is removed and biopsied, and if endometriosis is diagnosed, a proper course of treatment is then determined. **MRI** and sonogram (ultrasound) may also be used in select cases.

Sources:
1. National Institute of Child Health and Human Development, 2001.
2. National Women's Health Information Center, 1998.

Treatment options include:
- Birth control pills.
- Injections of the hormone **progesterone**.
- **NSAIDs** (nonsteriodal anti-inflammatory drugs), for pain management.
- Synthetic hormone therapy to temporarily stop periods and inhibit endometrium growth, often accompanied by "add-back therapy" to replace lost estrogen.
- In severe cases, a hysterectomy, or surgical removal of the uterus. Sometimes, the cervix and/or ovaries and fallopian tubes are also removed. (Symptoms may still return).

Common Sites of Endometriosis

Ectopic endometrial tissue can implant almost anywhere in the pelvic peritoneum. It can even invade distant sites, such as the lungs.

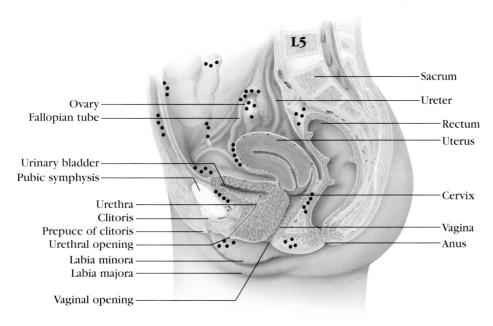

Normal Uterine and Ovarian Anatomy

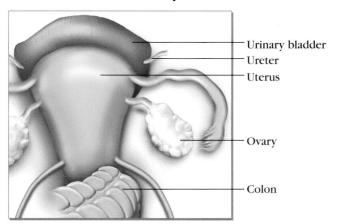

Endometriosis

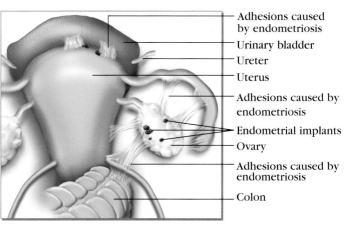

Infertility is the inability to conceive a pregnancy.

Only 20 percent of women who want to conceive become pregnant during the first ovulation cycle in which they try.[1]

Of the 80 percent of infertility cases with a diagnosed cause, about half are based at least partially on male factors.[2]

DETAILED DESCRIPTION

During ovulation, an egg is released from an ovary into the fallopian tube. If spermatozoa (sperm) travel through the fallopian tubes, they can penetrate an ovum (egg), causing fertilization. Once the egg is fertilized, it normally travels to the uterus, where it implants and continues to develop over the next nine months.

Infertility is a disease in which conception is not achieved after one year of twice-weekly unprotected intercourse. Infertility affects about 6.1 million people in the U.S., or about ten percent of the reproductive age population.[3]

RISK FACTORS

Pelvic Factors

- Tubal disorders caused by **pelvic inflammatory disease (PID)**, endometriosis, or prior pelvic surgery.
- Uterine disorders caused by benign **fibroid tumors** of the uterus, scarring from prior uterine surgery, or an abnormally shaped uterine cavity.

Ovulatory Factors

- Hormonal abnormalities including **polycystic ovarian syndrome**, **thyroid** abnormalities, and **pituitary** abnormalities.
- Age—Infertility becomes more pronounced after the age of 35.[4]
- Excessive exercise, drug and alcohol abuse, obesity, or being underweight.
- Other pre-existing medical problems.

Cervical Factors

- Abnormal cervical mucus.
- Prior cervical surgery.

Male Factors

- Absence of or low sperm production, which can be caused by lifestyle or environmental factors or by medical conditions.
- Inability to ejaculate.

SYMPTOMS & SIGNS

Fertility problems should be brought to the attention of a health care provider after one year of regular, unprotected sex. Women over the age of 30 may want to consult a health care provider after six months of attempting conception.

Sources:
1. U.S. Food and Drug Administration, 1997.
2. National Women's Health Information Center, 1998.
3. American Society of Reproductive Medicine, 2002.
4. American Society of Reproductive Medicine, 2002.

PREVENTION & MANAGEMENT

General habits that can maximize a woman's fertility include:
- Safe sex with as few partners as possible.
- Regular exercise.
- Maintenance of a healthy body weight.
- Caffeine intake of no more than 3 to 4 cups of coffee daily.
- Abstinence from illegal drugs.
- Abstinence from nicotine.
- Consultation with a health care provider for preconception counseling.

It is also important to avoid drinking alcohol because of the harm it could cause to a fetus.

Evaluation by a health care provider will help determine the cause of the infertility. Treatment needs to be tailored to the specific cause.

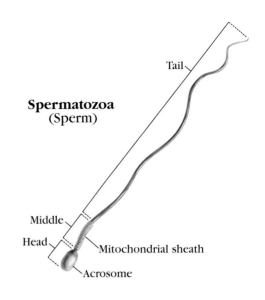

Spermatozoa
(Sperm)

Fertilization and Implantation

During monthly ovulation, an ovum is released from the ovary into the fallopian tube, where it travels toward the uterus. If present, sperm from the male move through the fallopian tube, where they meet the ovum.

If a sperm penetrates the ovum, fertilization occurs and the ovum is called a zygote. The zygote continues to travel toward the uterus, dividing many times until it becomes a blastocyst. There it implants in the uterine lining and will continue to develop over the next nine months.

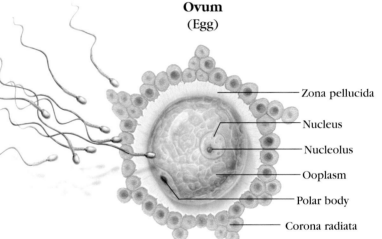

Ovum
(Egg)

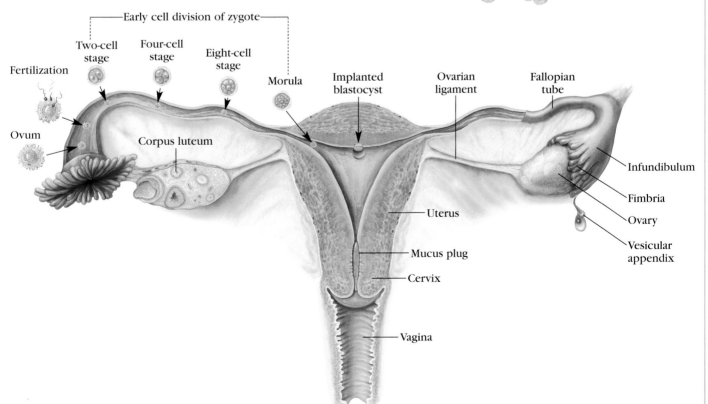

58

Pregnancy is the condition of a female after conception until the birth of the baby.

Drinking alcohol during pregnancy is the most preventable cause of mental retardation. Smoking during pregnancy is associated with higher rates of miscarriage and premature birth.[1]

Good nutrition is a crucial step in having a healthy baby. A pregnancy takes about 300 extra calories a day to maintain, and an average-sized woman can expect to gain between 25 and 35 pounds overall.[2]

DETAILED DESCRIPTION

A normal, full-term pregnancy lasts between 37 and 42 weeks. Pregnancy is divided into three segments called trimesters. During each trimester, a woman's body undergoes substantial changes as the fetus develops.

RISK FACTORS

Factors that can contribute to a high-risk pregnancy include:
• Medical conditions such as diabetes, hypertension, **epilepsy**, kidney disease, heart disease, a genetic disease, or a sexually transmitted disease.
• History of tubal disease or of pain and/or bleeding in the first trimester. These are risk factors for an ectopic pregnancy (a pregnancy that occurs outside the uterus).
• Multiple gestation (twins, triplets, etc.).
• Pregnancy complications including **gestational diabetes** and **pre-eclampsia**.
• Previous premature delivery or pre-term labor.
• Reproductive structural abnormalities.

SYMPTOMS & SIGNS

A woman undergoes a vast array of physical, hormonal, and emotional changes over the course of a pregnancy, including weight gain. Others include:
• Absence of menstruation.
• Nausea and vomiting.
• Breast tenderness.
• Indigestion.
• Lower back pain.
• Constipation and/or hemorrhoids.
• Fatigue.
• Increased urination.
• Skin changes, such as patches of darker skin on the face, stretch marks, or a dark line that runs from the navel to the pubic hair.
• Emotional changes, such as mood swings or weepiness. For an in-depth discussion of the emotional issues facing new mothers, please refer to the "Emotional Wellness" section.

Lower abdominal pain and vaginal bleeding are not normal in pregnancy and should always be brought to the attention of a health care provider.

PREVENTION & MANAGEMENT

General habits that increase chances for a healthy pregnancy include:
• Pre-conception counseling to assess potential risks.
• Good prenatal care with regular medical check-ups.
• A healthy lifestyle including exercise (with doctor's approval); eating a well-balanced diet; and avoiding drugs, tobacco, and alcohol.
• Avoidance of all medications not approved by the health care provider.
• Taking prenatal vitamins, especially folic acid, while trying to conceive and during pregnancy.

Trimester and Fetal Development

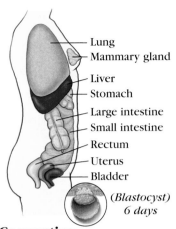

Lung
Mammary gland
Liver
Stomach
Large intestine
Small intestine
Rectum
Uterus
Bladder

(Blastocyst)
6 days

Conception

In the days immediately following conception, there is little change in the appearance of the body or position of organs.

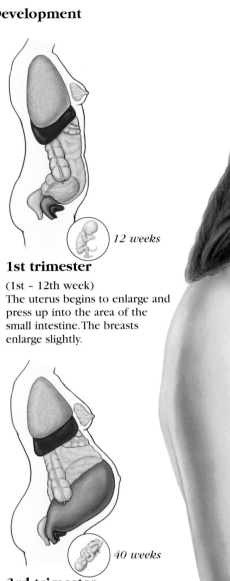

12 weeks

1st trimester

(1st – 12th week)
The uterus begins to enlarge and press up into the area of the small intestine. The breasts enlarge slightly.

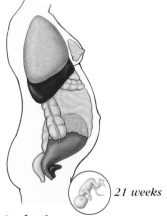

21 weeks

2nd trimester

(13th – 24th week)
The uterus continues to enlarge and press upward toward the small intestine, making urination more frequent.

40 weeks

3rd trimester

(25th – 40th week)
During this stage, the uterus presses down on the bladder, and the upward expansion of the uterus on the intestines puts pressure on the stomach, liver and lungs.

Mammary Glands

As a result of hormonal activity, the breasts may double in size during pregnancy. During this time fatty tissue is largely replaced by glandular tissue, and the mammary glands become capable of secreting milk.

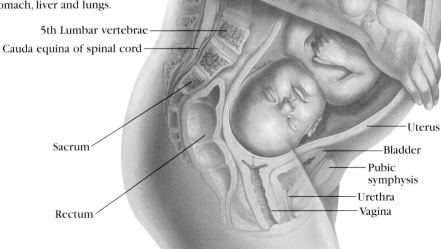

Gland lobule

Lactiferous sinus and duct

Placenta

Umbilical cord

5th Lumbar vertebrae
Cauda equina of spinal cord

Uterus
Bladder
Pubic symphysis
Urethra
Vagina

Sacrum

Rectum

Sources:
1. U.S. Food and Drug Administration, 1997.
2. U.S. Food and Drug Administration, 1999.

Labor is a physiological process that culminates in the birth of a child.

American women are having more children than at any other time in the last 30 years. The average American woman gives birth to two children over the course of a lifetime.[1]

Nearly 23 percent of births require cesarean delivery.[2]

DETAILED DESCRIPTION

Between weeks 37 and 42 of a normal pregnancy, a woman will go into labor and give birth. Although each woman has a different childbirth experience, labor and delivery can be divided into three distinct stages:

1. *First stage*—Uterine muscles begin to contract at regular intervals. The contractions cause the cervix of the uterus to dilate (open) and efface (thin out). This stage ends once the cervix has dilated to 10 centimeters.
2. *Second stage*—Forceful uterine contractions and maternal effort push the fetus from the uterus through the birth canal. This stage ends with the birth of the child.
3. *Third stage*—The placenta separates from the uterine wall and is expelled.

RISK FACTORS

Risk factors that can complicate natural labor and delivery include:
- Pre-existing medical conditions.
- Previous cesarean section delivery.
- Multiple gestation (twins, triplets, etc.).
- **Breech presentation**.
- Post-term pregnancy (after 42 weeks).
- Pre-term labor (prior to 37 weeks).
- **Gestational diabetes**.

Risk factors can put a woman at increased risk of having a cesarean delivery. A cesarean delivery occurs when a baby is delivered through a surgical incision made in the uterus. Conditions for a cesarean delivery include:
- Prolonged labor.
- A baby that is too large to pass through the pelvis.
- Complications with the baby, such as irregular heartbeat or lack of oxygen.
- Breech presentation.
- Previous cesarean delivery.

SYMPTOMS & SIGNS

It is not known precisely what triggers the onset of labor. For most women, the signs of labor include:
- Strong, regular contractions.
- Blood-tinged or mucus discharge, caused by cervical dilation and effacement.
- Breaking of the amniotic sac (common term: "water breaks").

You should contact your health care provider when any of these signs occur.

PREVENTION & MANAGEMENT

Prenatal care and birthing classes can help educate you and your partner on what to expect during labor and how to make the experience more enjoyable.

Sources:
1. Centers for Disease Control, 2002.
2. Centers for Disease Control, 2002.

Three Stages of Labor

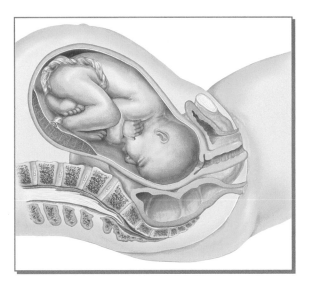

1 **First stage–Dilation**

Uterine muscles begin to contract at regular intervals. As the time between contractions becomes shorter, the contractions become longer and more intense. During this cycle the cervix of the uterus dilates. As the cervix dilates, the mucus plug is discharged.

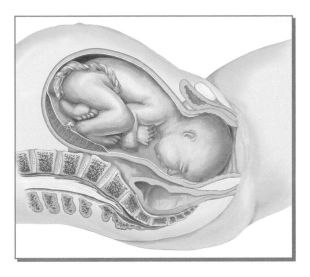

2 **Second stage–Childbirth**

Forceful uterine contractions push the fetus from the uterus through the birth canal.

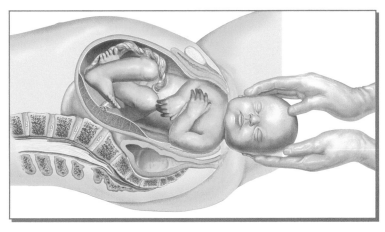

Delivery of the head and rotation.

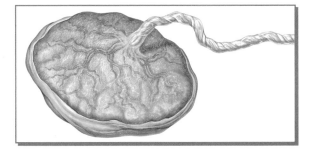

3 **Third stage–Afterbirth**

After the birth, the placenta separates from the uterine wall and is expelled.

Menopause refers to the complete cessation of a woman's menstrual cycle.

More than one third of women in the United States, about 36 million, have been through menopause. With a life expectancy of about 81 years, a 50-year-old-woman can expect to live more than one third of her life after menopause.[1]

Many post-menopausal women mistakenly believe that regular gynecological exams are no longer necessary. In truth, it is at precisely this point in life when women are at higher risk for cancers of the reproductive system, and other gynecological problems.[2]

DETAILED DESCRIPTION

The word *menopause* is derived from the Greek words *men*, which means "monthly," and *pauses*, which means "ending." Literally, menopause refers to the last spontaneous menstrual period and occurs as a natural result of loss of ovarian function. This end to the menstrual cycle means the end of **ovulation**, the end of menstrual periods, and the end of the possibility of pregnancy.

Menopause occurs any time between the ages of 40 and 60, usually beginning at around age 50. For many women, the signs of menopause occur for a period of time before menopause has technically taken place. Perimenopause refers to the time in a woman's life from the first sign of menstrual irregularity to one year after the last menstrual period.

SYMPTOMS & SIGNS

While some menopausal women notice no changes other than the cessation of menstrual periods, others go through a variety of physical and/or emotional changes. During menopause, estrogen production decreases; postmenopausal **estrogen** levels are about 75 percent lower than during the reproductive years. Changes experienced during perimenopause and menopause are the body's response to this decrease:

- Irregular periods (perimenopause) or no periods (menopause).
- Thinning of genital-urinary tissues, which may lead to painful intercourse.
- Hot flashes.
- Night sweats and insomnia.
- Mood disturbances.

PREVENTION & MANAGEMENT

Health concerns associated with menopause include:

- Increased osteoporosis risk.
- Increased heart disease risk.
- Increased high blood pressure risk.
- Increased high cholesterol risk.
- Weight gain.

Treatment options to manage the symptoms and long-term effects of menopause include **hormone replacement therapy (HRT)**, diet, and exercise. Perimenopausal women should take advantage of preventive options such as breast exams, **mammography**, **colonoscopy**, and cholesterol checks.

For a more in-depth discussion of menopause, please refer to the "Healthy Aging" section.

Sources:
1. National Women's Health Information Center, 1999.
2. National Women's Health Information Center, 1999.

Ovarian Aging

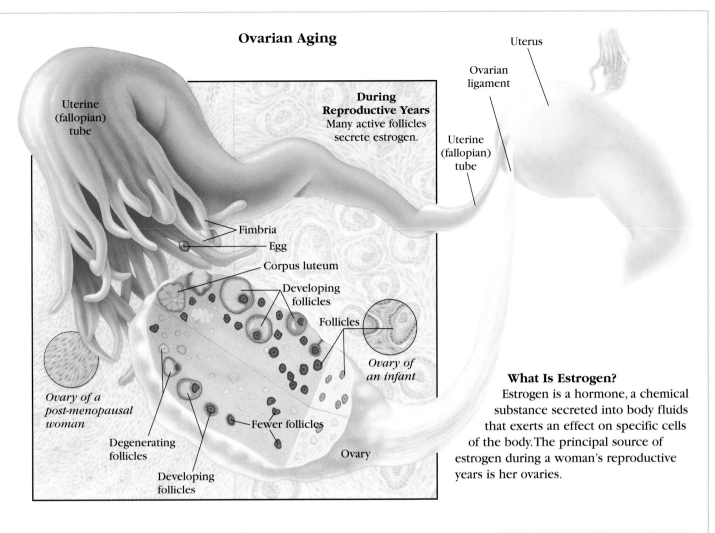

Uterine (fallopian) tube

During Reproductive Years
Many active follicles secrete estrogen.

Uterus

Ovarian ligament

Uterine (fallopian) tube

Fimbria

Egg

Corpus luteum

Developing follicles

Follicles

Ovary of an infant

Ovary of a post-menopausal woman

Degenerating follicles

Fewer follicles

Developing follicles

Ovary

What Is Estrogen?
Estrogen is a hormone, a chemical substance secreted into body fluids that exerts an effect on specific cells of the body. The principal source of estrogen during a woman's reproductive years is her ovaries.

Symptoms of Menopause

Irregular Menstruation
Irregularity of menstrual periods is the earliest, most common symptom of menopause.

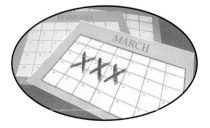

Painful Intercourse
Lower estrogen levels can cause thinning of vaginal tissues and a decrease in lubricating fluid, leading to uncomfortable or painful intercourse.

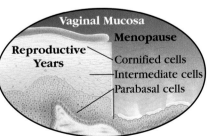

Vaginal Mucosa

Menopause

Reproductive Years

Cornified cells
Intermediate cells
Parabasal cells

Hot Flashes, Night Sweats and Insomnia
Hot flashes, a warm feeling in the face and neck that sometimes spreads to the back or chest, may happen throughout the day and night, causing discomfort and interfering with restful sleep. Hot flashes are caused by low estrogen levels but are not completely understood. Although hot flashes are uncomfortable, they are not dangerous and are usually unnoticed by others.

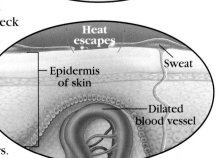

Heat escapes

Sweat

Epidermis of skin

Dilated blood vessel

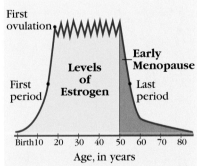

First ovulation

First period

Levels of Estrogen

Early Menopause

Last period

Birth 10 20 30 40 50 60 70 80

Age, in years

At the onset of menopause, many of the follicles in the ovaries have either been "used up" or have degenerated over time. Estrogen production goes down as the number of follicles decreases. When estrogen levels fall below a critical value, ovulation cannot occur consistently, and menstrual periods become irregular. Eventually, all follicles degenerate and reproductive cycles stop altogether.

An ovarian cyst is a fluid-filled sac that forms on the ovary.

Post-menopausal women who develop ovarian cysts have a greater likelihood of developing ovarian cancer and require more aggressive, immediate medical treatment.[1]

An estimated 5 to 10 percent of women of childbearing age have polycystic ovarian syndrome (PCOS).[2]

DETAILED DESCRIPTION

Ovarian cysts are fluid-filled sacs that can form on or within the ovary under a variety of conditions. They can range in size from a pea to a grapefruit and can affect either or both of the ovaries. The cysts are more common during the childbearing years, and although most are benign (noncancerous), it is important to seek medical attention if a cyst is suspected.

There are several types of ovarian cysts:

- *Functional cysts*—Ovarian cysts that occur as a result of normal changes during the menstrual cycle and generally disappear on their own after one to three months. Follicular cysts, a type of functional cyst, occur when the follicle within the ovary matures but fails to release an egg. The follicle continues to grow but generally disappears within three months.
- *Endometriomas*—Cysts associated with endometriosis which are composed of tissue similar to the tissue that lines the uterus. The tissue implants itself in the ovary and grows to form a cyst.
- *Cystadenomas*—Benign ovarian tumors that develop from surface cells on the ovary. Cystadenomas are normally small but can become quite large and may need to be removed.
- *Dermoid cysts*—Ovarian cysts composed of different kinds of tissue such as hair, teeth, or bone.
- *Multiple Cysts*—Occurs when multiple cysts develop, causing the ovaries to swell. Usually caused by a condition called **polycystic ovary syndrome (PCOS)**.

RISK FACTORS

Women in their childbearing years have the greatest risk of developing an ovarian cyst.

SYMPTOMS & SIGNS

Ovarian cysts range greatly in size and in the severity of the symptoms they produce. Some women may never know they have an ovarian cyst, because the symptoms are not unique to cysts. Possible symptoms include:

- Severe pain in the lower abdomen.
- Irregular or lack of menstrual periods.
- Dull ache and/or swelling in the lower abdomen.
- Pain during intercourse.

PREVENTION & MANAGEMENT

Oral contraceptives may be used for prevention of some functional cysts.

Methods of managing existing cysts are based on the cyst's size, symptoms, and appearance (as seen on a sonogram, or ultrasound). A physician may simply monitor small, **asymptomatic** cysts that appear benign on a sonogram. Cysts that do not go away after several months or that increase in size or pain may need to be removed surgically. Cysts that occur after menopause are more likely to be surgically removed because of the higher risk of being cancerous.

Normal Uterine and Fallopian Anatomy

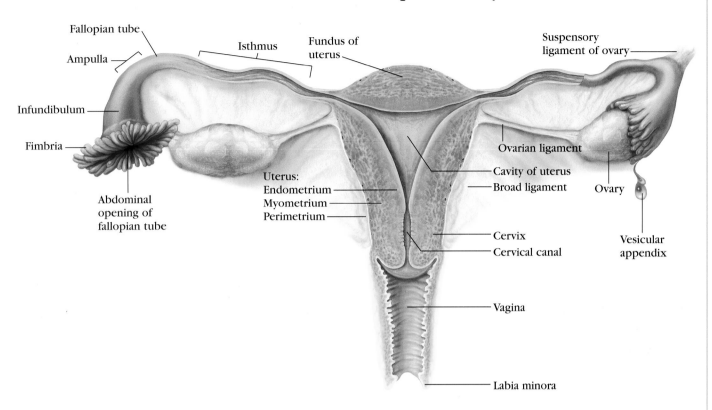

Fallopian tube

Ampulla

Infundibulum

Fimbria

Abdominal opening of fallopian tube

Isthmus

Fundus of uterus

Suspensory ligament of ovary

Ovarian ligament

Cavity of uterus

Broad ligament

Ovary

Uterus:
Endometrium
Myometrium
Perimetrium

Cervix

Cervical canal

Vesicular appendix

Vagina

Labia minora

Follicular Cyst

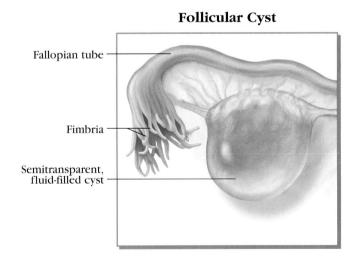

Fallopian tube

Fimbria

Semitransparent, fluid-filled cyst

Dermoid Cyst

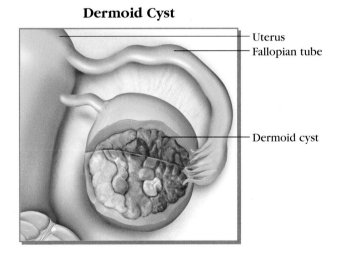

Uterus

Fallopian tube

Dermoid cyst

Sources:
1. National Women's Health Information Center, 2001.
2. National Women's Health Information Center, 2001.

Premenstrual syndrome, or PMS, is a pattern of physical and emotional symptoms experienced in the last 5 to 15 days of each menstrual cycle.

Research suggests that as many as 75 percent of menstruating women have some premenstrual syndrome symptoms.[1]

An estimated 3 to 4 percent of women suffer severe premenstrual symptoms that significantly interfere with work and social functioning. This impairing form of premenstrual syndrome, also called premenstrual dysphoric disorder (PMDD), appears to be the body's abnormal response to normal hormone changes.[2]

DETAILED DESCRIPTION

Premenstrual syndrome (PMS) includes a wide range of physical and emotional changes experienced by women in the days preceding their period. PMS symptoms are predictable, in that they occur before every menstrual cycle. Symptoms generally end abruptly once the period begins.

Although up to 75 percent of women have premenstrual symptoms,[3] not all experience premenstrual syndrome. Women who have mild or isolated symptoms associated with their menstrual cycle do not suffer from PMS. Symptoms that are severe enough to interfere with normal activities are considered to be indications of PMS. Women who experience symptoms in a predictable manner before each monthly period are considered to have PMS.

RISK FACTORS

The causes of PMS are not known. It is thought to result from hormonal changes, but it also may be related to chemical changes in the brain. Factors that can aggravate PMS include poor diet, stress, alcohol use, and caffeine intake.

SYMPTOMS & SIGNS

PMS includes a wide range of potential symptoms. The following are the most common:

- Bloating and fluid retention.
- Breast tenderness.
- Increased emotional sensitivity.
- Food cravings or changes in appetite.
- Sleeping problems.
- Headaches.
- Nausea or vomiting.
- Cramps.
- Joint or muscle aches.

In order for a health care provider to diagnose PMS, the pattern and severity of symptoms must be determined. If you think you have PMS, keep track of premenstrual symptoms for two or three menstrual cycles. Note when the symptoms begin and end and how severe you consider them to be. This will help your health care provider determine whether you have PMS.

Sources:
1. National Women's Health Information Center, 1998.
2. National Institute of Mental Health, 2001.
3. National Women's Health Information Center, 1998.

PREVENTION & MANAGEMENT

Lifestyle choices that may help minimize PMS symptoms:
- Take daily calcium supplements of 1,200 milligrams (mg).
- Take daily magnesium supplements of 200 mg.
- Limit salt intake to reduce water retention.
- Limit alcohol and caffeine intake.
- Eat a well-balanced diet.
- Exercise regularly.
- Get plenty of sleep.
- Practice relaxation techniques.
- Seek supportive therapy.

PMS is managed through a combination of lifestyle changes and, in more severe cases, medications, which could include:
- Anti-depressants.
- **Oral contraceptives**.
- Over-the-counter **Nonsteroidal Anti-Inflammatory Drugs (NSAIDS)**, such as ibuprofen.

Menstrual Cycle

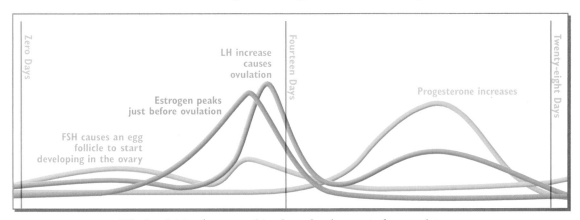

Hormone Changes During the Menstrual Cycle

LH= Luteinizing hormone: Stimulates development of corpus luteum.
FSH= Follicle-stimulating hormone: Stimulates growth of the follicle in the ovary.

Sexually transmitted diseases (STDs) are infections transmitted primarily through unprotected sexual intercourse with an infected partner.

Young women have a higher chance of getting an STD than older women.[1]

HPVs, or human papillomaviruses, are the leading cause of cervical cancer.[2]

DETAILED DESCRIPTION

Sexually transmitted diseases (STDs) affect 13 million Americans each year.[3] STDs pose significant health concerns for women in particular. Women are at a greater risk than men for developing an STD because the vagina is more conducive to disease growth than the male reproductive organs. Once an STD has been contracted, women experience more health problems that are more severe, in comparison to men. The symptoms of an STD are often not apparent because they occur inside the vagina. The risks associated with prolonged infection with an STD involve a variety of health complications, including infertility. Pregnant women with STDs are at an additional risk, since they can transmit the disease to their unborn children. STDs also increase the risk of **miscarriage**, premature birth, and **stillbirth**.

RISK FACTORS

Some STDs can be transmitted through oral sex. Other risk factors associated with STDs include:
- A history of multiple sexual partners.
- Illicit drug use.
- Age—nearly two-thirds of all STDs occur in people younger than 25 years old.[4]
- Sexual intercourse before age 16.
- Previous STD.

SYMPTOMS & SIGNS

Many STDs present no symptoms at all, which makes regular testing by a gynecologist important. Following are the most common STDs and the symptoms associated with them:
- *Chlamydia*—the most common STD and the most common cause of **pelvic inflammatory disease (PID)**, can lead to infertility. Chlamydia often produces no symptoms, making it difficult to diagnose. Potential symptoms include abnormal vaginal discharge, burning sensation during urination, pain during intercourse, and bleeding after intercourse.
- *Gonorrhea*—the most prevalent STD among sexually active teenage girls. Most women who are infected with gonorrhea have no symptoms. The most common consequence of gonorrhea is the development of pelvic inflammatory disease (PID), resulting in infertility in as many as 10 percent of women affected.[5] Potential symptoms include a yellow-green discharge from the vagina or rectum and a burning sensation during urination.
- *Genital warts*—a common STD caused by HPVs, or the human papilloma viruses (a group of more than 100 viruses). Symptoms include painless, white warts on the genitals, anus, or throat. No cure exists for genital warts. In addition to genital warts, certain high-risk types of HPV cause cervical cancer and other genital cancers.
- *Herpes simplex*—a highly contagious STD that can be transmitted through skin-to-skin contact. Symptoms include blister-like sores on the genitals or mouth. No cure exists for herpes.

- *HIV/AIDS*—acquired immunodeficiency syndrome (AIDS) is a disease that is caused by the human immunodeficiency virus (HIV), which eventually destroys the body's immune system. Transmission of the virus primarily occurs during sexual activity and by sharing needles used to inject **intravenous** drugs. The presence of other STDs increases the likelihood of HIV infection after unprotected intercourse with an infected partner. Symptoms of HIV infection include flu-like symptoms and swollen lymph nodes. Some people with HIV experience no symptoms for many years. No cure exists for HIV or AIDS.
- *Trichomoniasis*—an extremely common STD that can cause pain during urination and a frothy green or gray discharge.
- *Syphilis*—a potentially fatal, yet rare, STD that usually begins with a raised sore in the genital area. If left untreated, syphilis can lead to life-threatening complications and even death.

PREVENTION & MANAGEMENT

The only way to prevent STDs is through sexual abstinence, but other practices can help reduce the risk of contracting an STD:
- Use a condom every time you have sexual intercourse or oral sex.
- Limit number of sexual partners over your lifetime.
- Have a mutually monogamous sexual relationship with an uninfected partner.
- Do not douche; douching disrupts healthy bacteria levels in the vagina.
- Use clean needles if injecting intravenous drugs.

Regular, yearly visits to the gynecologist are essential in the treatment of STDs. Because many STDs do not cause symptoms early on, regular screenings are required if you are sexually active. If an STD is detected, your health care provider will determine the best course of treatment. Some STDs have no cure, although the symptoms can be managed.

Common Sites Affected by STDs

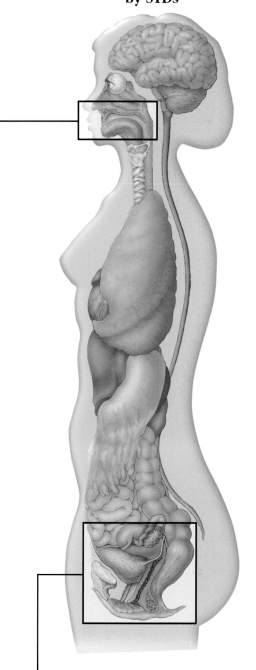

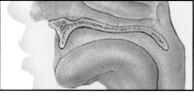

- Blisters in Oral Cavity.

- Pelvic Scarring.
- Genital Damage.
- Cervical Cancer.
- Pelvic Inflammatory Disease.
- Urethritis (Inflammatory of Urethra).
- Itching.
- Rashes.
- Swollen Lymph Nodes.
- Childbearing Problems.
- Warts.

Sources:
1. National Women's Health Information Center, 1999.
2. National Cancer Institute, 2001.
3. National Institutes of Health, 1999.
4. National Institute of Allergy and Infectious Diseases, 1999.
5. National Women's Health Information Center, 1998.

Vaginitis is an irritation, swelling, or redness of the vagina and vulva that can be caused by an irritant or infection.

Nearly 75 percent of all women will experience a yeast infection at some point in their lives.[1]

Trichomoniasis, or "trich," is a common sexually transmitted disease that affects 2 to 3 million Americans yearly.[2]

DETAILED DESCRIPTION

Vaginitis is a common gynecological problem that affects women of all ages. It is one of the most frequent reasons for women to visit a gynecologist. Vaginitis can be caused by anything that upsets the natural ecosystem of the vagina. A visit to your health care provider will help determine the cause and correct treatment of vaginitis.

Common Forms of Vaginitis

- *Bacterial vaginosis*—the most common form of vaginitis in American women. It is caused by an overgrowth of bacteria normally present in the vagina.
- *Yeast infection*, or *vulvovaginal candidiasis*—caused by the overgrowth of fungus in the vagina.
- *Trichomoniasis*—a sexually transmitted disease caused by a parasite introduced through unprotected intercourse.
- *Atrophic vaginitis*—occurs in women with low levels of **estrogen**, such as post-menopausal women, breastfeeding mothers, and women who have had their ovaries removed (which could accompany a **hysterectomy**). Low levels of estrogen can cause vaginal tissue to become dry and thin, increasing the risk of irritation.

RISK FACTORS

Risk factors for vaginitis include anything that might upset the natural vaginal ecosystem:

- Poor personal hygiene.
- Using too much soap.
- Wearing clothes that are too tight.
- Use of feminine deodorants, douches, and scented sanitary products.
- Use of certain medications (check drug information for side effects).
- Sexual intercourse.
- Stress.
- Change in sexual partners.
- Hormonal changes.
- Unprotected sex with someone infected with an STD.
- Pregnancy, recent childbirth, or menopause.
- Inadequate sleep.
- Poor nutrition.

SYMPTOMS & SIGNS

In addition to itching, burning, and redness of the vagina, other symptoms include:

- *Bacterial vaginosis*—thin vaginal discharge with a dark, dull-gray color and a fishy odor, especially following intercourse.
- *Yeast infection*—a cottage cheese–like discharge.
- *Trichomoniasis*—yellow-green or gray discharge, which can be frothy and have an odor; possible pain during urination.
- *Atrophic vaginitis*—vaginal dryness and burning; a feeling of pressure during sexual intercourse.

PREVENTION & MANAGEMENT

• Maintain good personal hygiene.
• Avoid scented feminine care products, especially douches.
• Wear underpants with a cotton crotch.
• Avoid tight-fitting clothing.
• Eat a well-balanced diet.
• Get plenty of rest.

It is important to report symptoms of vaginitis to your doctor, so that a proper diagnosis can be made. Many symptoms of vaginitis are similar to those of an STD. Treatments for vaginitis include:

• Over-the-counter or prescription creams.
• Antibiotics.
• Water-soluble lubricants.
• **Hormone replacement therapy (HRT)**.

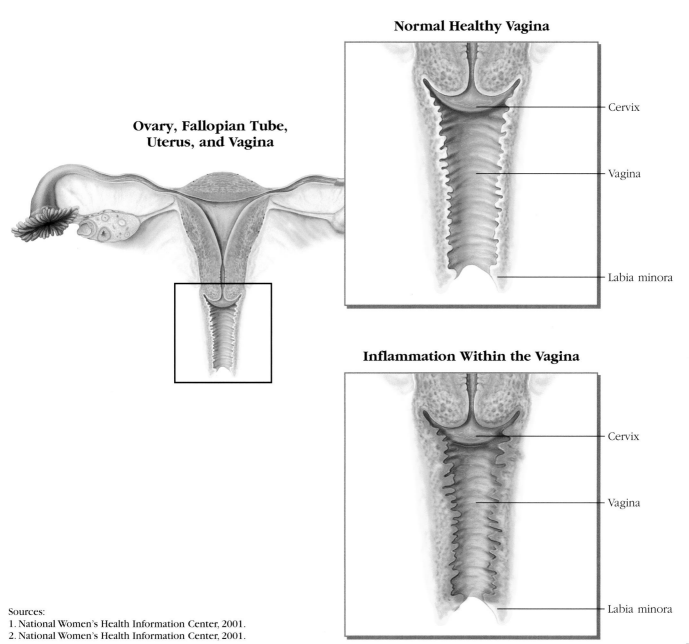

Ovary, Fallopian Tube, Uterus, and Vagina

Normal Healthy Vagina

Cervix

Vagina

Labia minora

Inflammation Within the Vagina

Cervix

Vagina

Labia minora

Sources:
1. National Women's Health Information Center, 2001.
2. National Women's Health Information Center, 2001.

Cancers

"Nothing in life is to be feared. It is only to be understood."
Marie Curie

Women experience a unique set of cancers that are directly related to their reproductive system, as well as the same nonreproductive cancers that men may have. A woman's lifelong cancer risk varies according to fluctuating hormone levels, advancing age, and other factors. By learning more about the common signs of cancer, as well as ways to prevent it, women can increase rates of survival and decrease cancer risk. If caught early, cancer can become a catalyst for healthier living and enhanced wellness.

Topics:
 Understanding Cancer
 Breast Cancer
 Colorectal Cancer
 Endometrial Cancer
 Lung Cancer
 Ovarian Cancer
 Skin Cancer

Cancer is the uncontrolled growth of abnormal cells in the body.

Of all cancers, lung cancer is the leading killer of women and accounts for 25 percent of women's cancer deaths each year.[1]

Several cancers are associated with obesity: breast, endometrium, colon, kidney, esophagus, stomach, and gallbladder. Some studies have also reported links between obesity and cancers of the prostate, ovaries, and pancreas.[2]

DETAILED DESCRIPTION

Cancer is the second leading cause of death in the United States.[3] Cancer cells divide rapidly and tend to be aggressive. Cancer that begins in a particular organ, such as the breast or skin, can invade nearby tissues and spread to other areas of the body. There are three ways in which cancer cells may move to other tissues: via the bloodstream, through the **lymphatic system**, or by shedding and seeding. Shedding occurs when cancer penetrates an organ or tissue and spreads into a body cavity, where it tends to seed (form new tumors).

RISK FACTORS

Experts do not think that there is one single cause of cancer. Rather, cancer seems to result from a complex mix of factors related to heredity, lifestyle, and environment. Risk factors may include:

• Advancing age.
• Smoking or regular exposure to tobacco smoke.
• Unhealthy dietary habits. For instance, some research links a high-fat diet to cancers of the colon, uterus, and prostate.
• Heavy alcohol use.
• Sun exposure.
• Very high doses of ionizing radiation from x-rays, radiation therapy, and other sources.
• Exposure to substances such as certain chemicals, metals, or pesticides.
• Conditions or treatments associated with high levels of exposure to estrogen.
• A history of cancer in close family members.
• Excess weight.

SYMPTOMS & SIGNS

Early detection is crucial to catching cancer when it is most treatable. Symptoms vary according to the type of cancer and may include the following:

• Change in bowel or bladder habits.
• A sore that does not heal.
• Unusual bleeding or discharge.
• Thickening or lump in the breast or elsewhere.
• Indigestion or difficulty swallowing.
• Obvious change in wart or mole.
• Nagging cough or hoarseness.
• Unexplained changes in weight.

Sources:
1. Women and Smoking: A Report of the Surgeon General, 2001.
2. National Cancer Institute, 2001.
3. National Vital Statistics, 2001.

PREVENTION & MANAGEMENT

The following lifestyle habits may offer protection against cancer:

• Eat a high-fiber, low-fat diet.
• Avoid excess alcohol.
• Maintain a healthy weight.
• Exercise regularly.
• Get regular cancer screenings.
• Quit smoking or don't start.
• Use sunscreen when in the sun.

Treatment for cancer depends on the type of cancer and many other factors. Options may include:

• Surgery to remove cancer.
• **Radiation**.
• **Chemotherapy**.
• **Hormonal therapy**.
• **Immunotherapy**.

Some patients with cancer may benefit from participating in cancer support groups. A hospital oncology department or cancer treatment center can provide information on these groups.

Cancer Incidence by Site

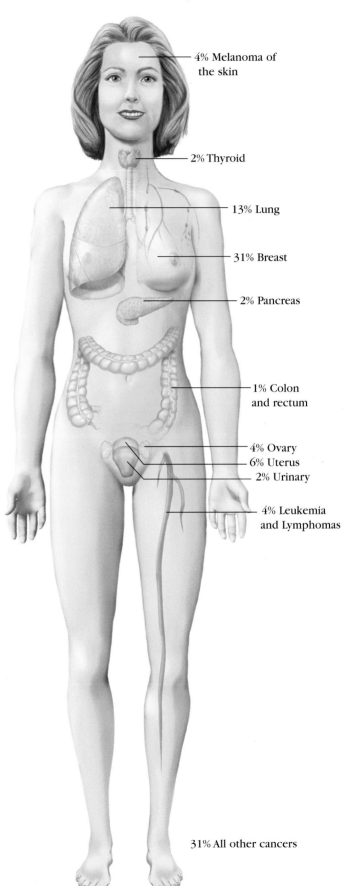

4% Melanoma of the skin

2% Thyroid

13% Lung

31% Breast

2% Pancreas

1% Colon and rectum

4% Ovary
6% Uterus
2% Urinary

4% Leukemia and Lymphomas

31% All other cancers

Cellular Progression

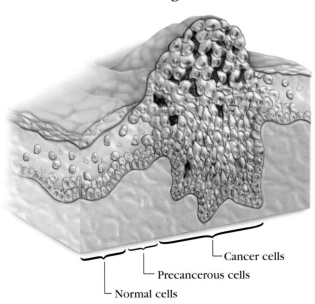

Cancer cells

Precancerous cells

Normal cells

76

Breast cancer is the uncontrolled growth of abnormal cells in the breast.

African American females have higher death rates from breast cancer than any other racial or ethnic group, even though Caucasian women have higher incidence rates. This disparity may be due to social factors rather than ethnicity.[1]

About 1 in 8 women in the United States (approximately 12.8 percent) will develop breast cancer during their lifetimes.[2]

DETAILED DESCRIPTION

Other than skin cancer, breast cancer is the most common type of cancer among women in the United States. More than 180,000 women are diagnosed with breast cancer each year.[3] Breast cancer may spread by way of the **lymphatic system** and/or bloodstream to the lungs, liver, bones, and other organs.

The most common category of breast cancer is ductal carcinoma, which begins in the lining of the ducts. Another less common category of breast cancer, lobular carcinoma, arises in the lobules of the breast.

Within the ductal carcinoma category, the two most common types of cancer are ductal carcinoma in situ (DCIS) and infiltrating ductal carcinoma (IDC). DCIS is breast cancer at its earliest stage, and is confined to the ducts that produce milk. IDC is breast cancer that has invaded the fatty tissue of the breast.

RISK FACTORS

The exact cause of breast cancer is not known. Risk factors include:
• Advancing age.
• Conditions associated with high levels of estrogen, such as early menstruation, late menopause, and no full-term pregnancies.
• First full-term pregnancy after age 30.
• Having a mother, sister, or daughter who has or had breast cancer, especially at a young age.
• Genetic mutations, such as BRCA1 and BRCA2, that are associated with breast and ovarian cancer. A blood test can reveal if a woman carries these genetic alterations.
• Menopausal obesity.

SYMPTOMS & SIGNS

Women should see a doctor if they detect any of the following symptoms:
• A lump or mass in or near the breast or in the underarm area.
• A change in breast shape or size.
• A change in the breast skin, such as dimpling, scaliness, or a change in color or temperature.
• Breast discharge or tenderness.
• The nipple pulled back into the breast.

There are several methods of detecting breast cancer including:
• Monthly breast self-exams.
• Annual breast exam by a trained health care provider
• Annual mammography starting at age 40, or according to your health care provider's recommendation.

Sources:
1. National Cancer Institute, 2002.
2. National Cancer Institute, 2001.
3. National Cancer Institute, 2002.

PREVENTION & MANAGEMENT

Women may be able to lower their risk of breast cancer with healthy habits, such as exercising regularly and limiting alcohol intake. Women who have a high risk of developing breast cancer may want to talk to a doctor about preventive medication or surgery. Studies show that the drug tamoxifen can reduce the risk of invasive breast cancer in high-risk women. Some high-risk women also choose to have their healthy breasts surgically removed to lower their risk of developing breast cancer in the future.

Women who develop breast cancer now have many treatment options, including:

- Surgery:
  - **Lumpectomy.**
  - **Partial mastectomy.**
  - **Total mastectomy.**
  - **Modified radical mastectomy.**
- **Chemotherapy.**
- **Radiation therapy.**
- **Hormonal therapy.**

Ductal Carcinoma in Situ (DCIS)

Common Sites of Breast Cancer Development

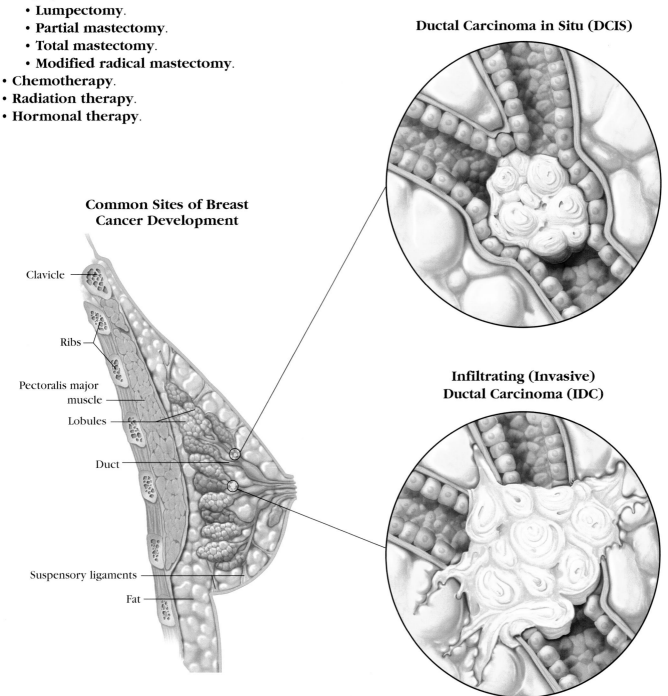

Clavicle

Ribs

Pectoralis major muscle

Lobules

Duct

Suspensory ligaments

Fat

Infiltrating (Invasive) Ductal Carcinoma (IDC)

Colorectal cancer is the uncontrolled growth of abnormal cells within the colon or rectum.

Together, cancers of the colon and rectum are among the most common cancers in the United States. They occur in both men and women and are most often found among people who are over the age of 50.[1]

Over 28,000 women die of colorectal cancer each year. Approximately 51,000 women per year are diagnosed with colon cancer. In addition, 16,500 new cases of rectal cancer are diagnosed in women each year.[2]

DETAILED DESCRIPTION

Colon cancer is the third leading cause of cancer in women.[3] Most of these cancers develop when benign (noncancerous) growths, or polyps, mutate into cancerous tumors. This is why it is necessary to remove polyps after they are found during colorectal cancer screenings.

RISK FACTORS

Most cases of colorectal cancer are diagnosed in people over age 50.[4] Risk factors besides advancing age include:

- A diet high in animal fats and low in fiber and/or calcium.
- A family history of colon cancer in parents, siblings, or children.
- A personal history of ulcerative colitis.
- A personal history of ovarian, uterine, or breast cancer.
- A known presence or prior history of colon polyps.

SYMPTOMS & SIGNS

Colorectal cancer may not cause any symptoms in the early stages. But the following signs should raise suspicion:

- Blood in the stool.
- Constipation, diarrhea, or other bowel changes lasting for ten days or longer.
- Unexplained abdominal pain and tenderness.
- Unexplained weight loss.
- Constant fatigue.
- Unexplained iron deficiency anemia.

PREVENTION & MANAGEMENT

Several screening tests are used to diagnose polyps and colorectal cancer, including the following:

- Fecal occult blood test, which is used to test for hidden blood in the stool.
- Sigmoidoscopy and/or colonoscopy, which involve examining the rectum and colon using a lighted instrument.
- Barium enema, or x-rays of the colon and rectum.

A diet that is rich in fiber and calcium, low in animal fats, and includes folic acid supplements may lower a woman's risk of colorectal cancer.

Treatment depends on the extent of disease and may include:
- Surgical removal of the tumor.
- Additional use of **chemotherapy**.
- Additional use of **radiation therapy**.
- **Immunotherapy**.

Sources:
1. Source: National Cancer Institute, 2002.
2. Source: National Institute of Health's Women's Health Initiative, 2002.
3. National Cancer Institute, 2001.
4. National Cancer Institute, 2002.

Types of Colorectal Cancer

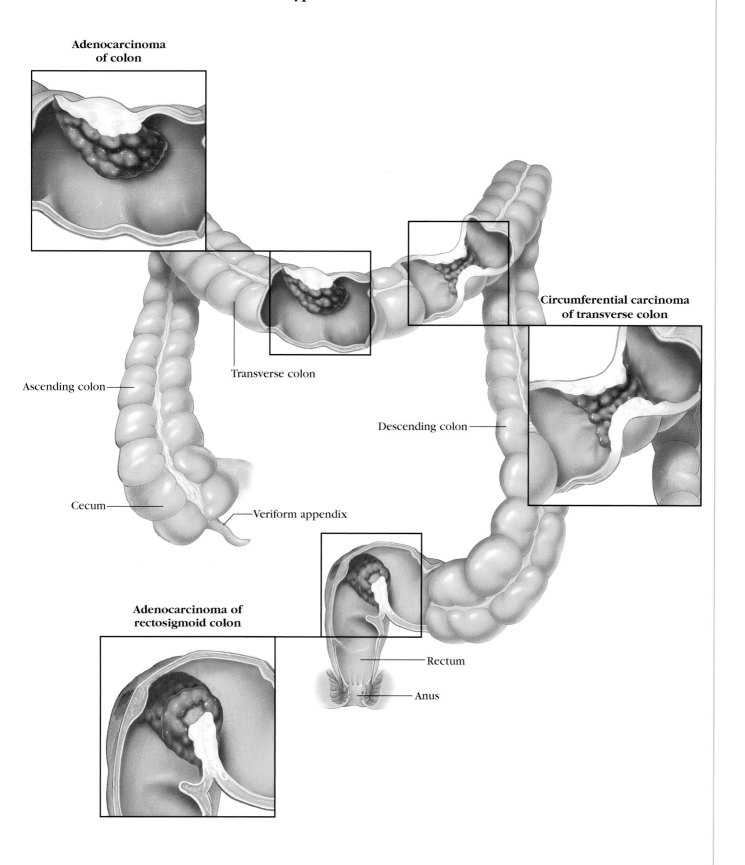

**Adenocarcinoma
of colon**

**Circumferential carcinoma
of transverse colon**

Transverse colon

Ascending colon

Descending colon

Cecum

Veriform appendix

**Adenocarcinoma of
rectosigmoid colon**

Rectum

Anus

Endometrial cancer is the uncontrolled growth of abnormal cells in the lining of the uterus.

Endometrial cancer is the most common reproductive cancer among women living in the United States.[1]

Abnormal uterine bleeding should not be considered a normal part of menopause. Always bring it to the attention of a health care provider to rule out a more serious condition, such as endometrial cancer.[2]

DETAILED DESCRIPTION

In the United States, endometrial cancer is the most common female reproductive cancer and accounts for six percent of all cancers in U.S. women.[3] Endometrial cancer, also known as uterine cancer, begins in the lining of the uterus called the endometrium. The cause of this cancer is currently unknown, but may be related to hormonal changes.

RISK FACTORS

- Age—postmenopausal women have a higher risk of developing endometrial cancer, but the disease can occur in younger women, too.
- A personal history of endometrial hyperplasia, or abnormal thickening of the uterine lining.
- Unopposed estrogen (estrogen taken without progesterone).
- Obesity.
- Use of the drug tamoxifen to treat breast cancer.
- A personal history of colorectal cancer.
- Race—Caucasian women are more likely than African-American women to get endometrial cancer.[4]
- An increased exposure to estrogen due to early menstruation, late menopause, or not giving birth to any children.

SYMPTOMS & SIGNS

A woman should see a doctor if she experiences any of the following symptoms:

- Abnormal vaginal bleeding or discharge.
- Any bleeding or spotting in postmenopause.
- Pelvic pain.
- Difficult or painful urination.
- Dyspareunia, or sharp pelvic pain during or after intercourse.

PREVENTION & MANAGEMENT

The following strategies may lower a woman's risk of endometrial cancer:

- Use of oral contraceptives.
- Childbirth.
- Maintenance of a healthy body weight.

A doctor may perform various tests to determine if a woman has endometrial cancer, including:

- Biopsy—the removal of a small amount of tissue from the uterine lining to examine under a microscope.
- D&C (dilation and curettage)—scraping away endometrial tissue for examination.
- Hysteroscopy—the visual instrumental inspection of the inside of the uterus.

Sources:
1. National Cancer Institute, 2002.
2. National Cancer Institute, 2001.
3. National Cancer Institute, 2002.
4. National Cancer Institute, 2002.

Treatment depends on the size of the tumor and many other factors. Options may include:

- Hysterectomy—surgery to remove the uterus. Ovaries, and fallopian tubes may be removed also.
- Removal of selected lymph nodes in the pelvis and lower abdomen.
- **Radiation therapy**.
- **Hormonal therapy**.

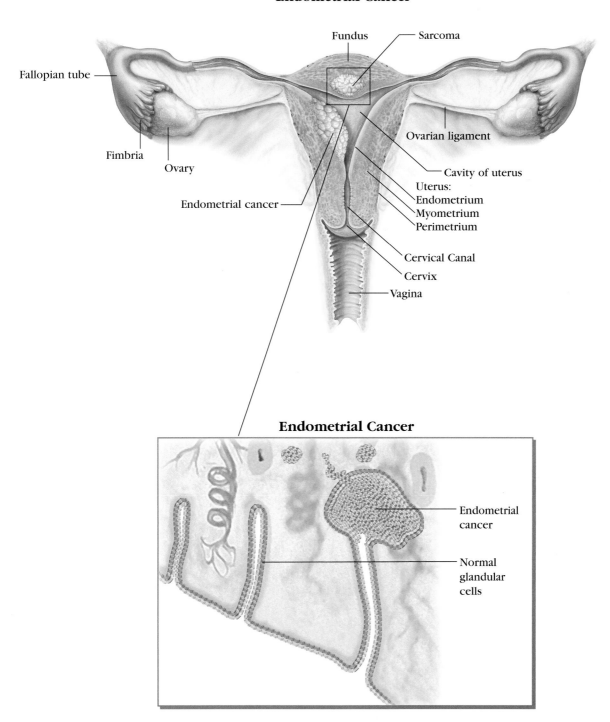

Progression of Endometrial Cancer

Fundus

Sarcoma

Fallopian tube

Fimbria

Ovary

Endometrial cancer

Ovarian ligament

Cavity of uterus

Uterus:
Endometrium
Myometrium
Perimetrium

Cervical Canal

Cervix

Vagina

Endometrial Cancer

Endometrial cancer

Normal glandular cells

Lung cancer is the uncontrolled growth of abnormal cells in the lungs.

In 1987, lung cancer surpassed breast cancer to become the leading cause of cancer death among U.S. women. In the year 2000, about 27,000 more women died of lung cancer (67,600) than breast cancer (40,800).[1]

Women who stop smoking greatly reduce their risk of dying prematurely. The relative benefits of smoking cessation are greater when women stop smoking at younger ages, but smoking cessation is beneficial at all ages.[2]

DETAILED DESCRIPTION

Lung cancer is the most preventable form of cancer. New cases of lung cancer appear to be on the rise among white and African American women due to increased rates of smoking.

There are two main types of lung cancer: small-cell and non–small-cell **carcinoma**. Non–small-cell lung cancer is far more prevalent and tends to spread more slowly than does small-cell lung cancer. Small-cell lung cancer is less common and is more likely to spread to other parts of the body than non–small-cell lung cancer is.

RISK FACTORS

Cigarette smoking is by far the most important risk factor for lung cancer. Other risk factors include:
• Cigar and pipe smoking.
• Exposure to second-hand smoke.
• Exposure to radon.
• Exposure to cancer-causing substances, such as asbestos.
• Air pollution. (*Note:* Although researchers have found a link with exposure to certain air pollutants, the relationship between lung cancer and air pollution is not clearly defined, and more research is being done.)

SYMPTOMS & SIGNS

Lung cancer may be present for many years with no symptoms. Common symptoms include:
• A persistent cough that worsens over time.
• Coughing up blood.
• Constant chest pain.
• Recurring pneumonia or bronchitis.
• Shortness of breath and wheezing.
• Swelling of the face and neck.
• Fatigue.
• Loss of appetite.
• Unexplained weight loss.

PREVENTION & MANAGEMENT

The single best way to prevent lung cancer is to not smoke or to stop smoking. Even someone who has been smoking for years can lower their risk of lung cancer by quitting.

To determine if a patient has lung cancer, a doctor may perform the following:
• A physical examination.
• A chest x-ray.
• A sputum cytology—a microscopic evaluation of mucus from the lungs.
• A biopsy—the removal of a small sample of lung tissue for examination.

Sources:
1. Women and Smoking: A Report of the Surgeon General, 2001.
2. Women and Smoking: A Report of the Surgeon General, 2001.

Treatment depends on the type and stage of lung cancer.
Options include:
- Surgical removal of the tumor, the part of the lung containing the tumor, or the entire lung.
- **Chemotherapy**.
- **Radiation therapy**.
- **Palliative therapy** to relieve symptoms, including **electrocautery**, therapy using lasers, and placement of a stent to keep the lung open and functioning.

Tumor Infiltration in Lung Cancer

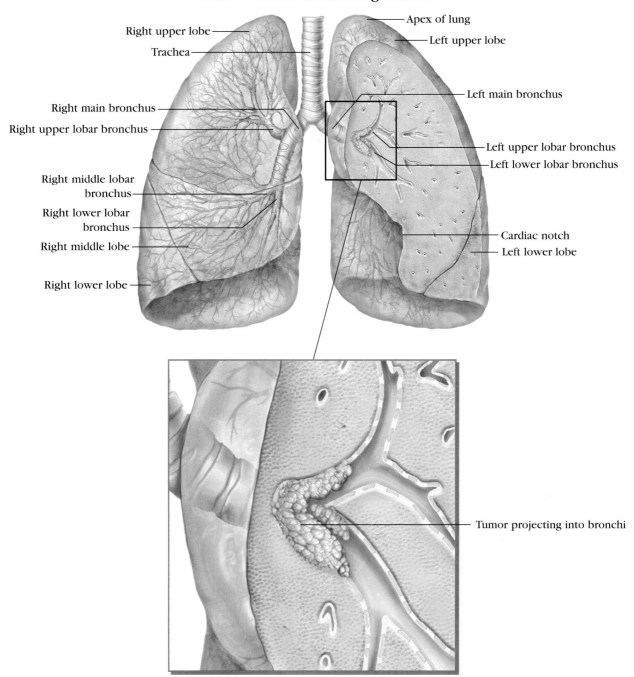

Right upper lobe

Trachea

Apex of lung

Left upper lobe

Right main bronchus

Right upper lobar bronchus

Left main bronchus

Left upper lobar bronchus

Left lower lobar bronchus

Right middle lobar bronchus

Right lower lobar bronchus

Right middle lobe

Cardiac notch

Left lower lobe

Right lower lobe

Tumor projecting into bronchi

Ovarian cancer is the uncontrolled growth of abnormal cells in the ovary.

About 1 in every 57 women in the United States will develop ovarian cancer. Most cases occur in women over the age of 50, but this disease can also affect younger women.[1]

Ovarian cancer is the fifth most commonly diagnosed cancer in women in the U.S. There are no proven methods of prevention, and it is often a rapidly fatal disease.[2]

DETAILED DESCRIPTION

Ovarian cancer is the most deadly of all the reproductive cancers because it is virtually undetectable until it has progressed to an advanced stage. Ovarian cancer begins either on the surface of the ovary, or more rarely, within the ovary itself. Ovarian cancer can spread to other parts of the abdomen (called shedding), where it forms new tumors (called seeding). Ovarian cancer can also spread by way of the **lymphatic system** or bloodstream to other areas of the body.

RISK FACTORS

Aging is one risk factor for ovarian cancer. Women are more likely to get the disease after age 50. Other risk factors include:
• A family history of ovarian cancer, especially if a woman's mother, sister, or daughter has had the disease.
• A personal or family history of breast or colon cancer.
• Genetic mutations, such as BRCA1 and BRCA2, that are associated with ovarian and breast cancer. A blood test can reveal if a woman carries these genetic alterations.
• Lack of full-term pregnancies associated with uninterrupted ovulation or undesired infertility. Women who have never had children are more likely to develop ovarian cancer than women who have had children.[3]

SYMPTOMS & SIGNS

Ovarian cancer is difficult to detect. Women often experience few or no symptoms until the disease has progressed to an advanced stage. Signs may include:
• Stomach bloating or discomfort.
• Feeling of fullness, even after little or no food.
• Persistent nausea or vomiting.
• Frequent urination or constipation.
• Loss of appetite.
• Unexplained weight gain or loss.

Experts are working hard to develop a screening test that can detect ovarian cancer before symptoms develop. Currently, doctors use a variety of tests to detect the disease, including pelvic exams and ultrasound.

PREVENTION & MANAGEMENT

The following strategies may offer some protection against ovarian cancer:
• Use of oral contraceptives.
• Childbirth and breastfeeding.
Some women who have a high risk of ovarian cancer choose to have their ovaries surgically removed before cancer has a chance to develop.

Sources:
1. National Cancer Institute, 2002.
2. National Cancer Institute, 2002.
3. National Cancer Institute, 2002.

Treatment options include:
- Surgical removal of the ovaries, uterus, fallopian tubes, and other affected tissues.
- If the cancer has spread, the surgeon may perform tumor debulking before chemotherapy or radiation therapy begins, which involves surgically removing as much of the tumor as possible.
- **Chemotherapy**.
- **Radiation therapy**, in select cases.

Ovarian Cancer

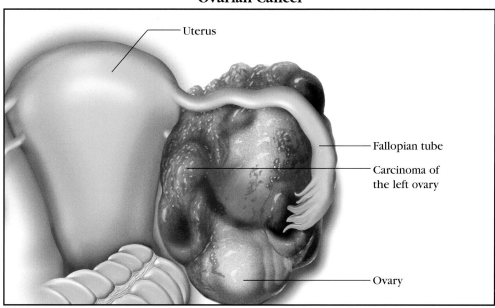

Uterus

Fallopian tube

Carcinoma of the left ovary

Ovary

Likely Metastatic Sites for Ovarian Cancer
Ovarian cancer can metastasize (spread) to almost any site.
Illustrated are the most common.

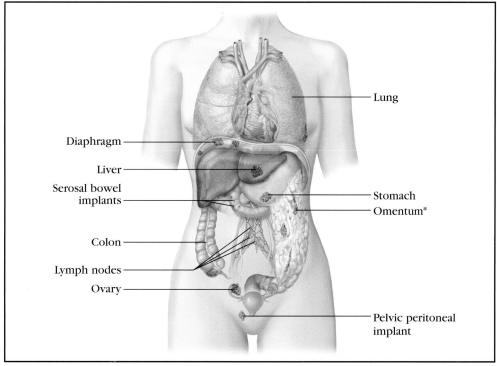

Lung

Diaphragm

Liver

Serosal bowel implants

Stomach

Omentum*

Colon

Lymph nodes

Ovary

Pelvic peritoneal implant

* Normally, the omentum extends from one side of the abdominal cavity to the other. For illustration purposes, this had been cut to reveal the anatomical structures that lie underneath.

Skin cancer is the uncontrolled growth of abnormal cells in a layer of the skin.

In women, the incidence of melanoma, the most serious form of skin cancer, is rising at a rate second only to lung cancer.[1]

According to current estimates, 40 to 50 percent of Americans who live to age 65 will have skin cancer at least once.[2]

DETAILED DESCRIPTION

In the United States, skin cancer is the most common type of cancer for both men and women. It normally results from prolonged, unprotected exposure to the sun.

The most common forms of skin cancer are basal-cell and squamous-cell carcinomas. Both occur in the top layer of the skin, called the epidermis. Basal-cell is more common than squamous-cell carcinoma, accounting for 90 percent of all skin cancers in the United States[3]. Basal- and squamous-cell cancers rarely spread to other parts of the body, but squamous-cell does so more often than basal-cell carcinoma.

Melanoma is the most serious form of skin cancer. It occurs in the cells of the skin that produce pigment, which gives skin its color. If left untreated, melanoma can spread to the lymph nodes and other parts of the body.

RISK FACTORS

Sun exposure is the main cause of skin cancer. Other risk factors include:
• A history of sunburns early in life.
• Use of sunlamps or tanning booths.
• Living in sunny climates or at high altitudes.
• Fair skin or freckles.
• A family history of skin cancer.
• Having abnormal-looking moles or a large number of moles.

SYMPTOMS & SIGNS

A doctor should be consulted immediately if there are any unusual growths or changes to the skin. Signs of skin cancer include:
• A firm, red lump.
• A small, smooth, shiny, pale, or waxy lump.
• A lump that bleeds or develops a crust.
• A growth or sore that doesn't heal.
• Any change in the size, shape, or color of a mole – look for the ABCD warning signs:
    • **A**symmetry: The shape of one half doesn't match the other half.
    • **B**orders: The edges are often irregular.
    • **C**olor: The color is uneven, and various colors, such as black, brown, or tan, may be present.
    • **D**iameter: Moles usually increase in size.

Also, a physician should be consulted if a flat, scaly patch on the skin that is red or brown develops. This may be a sign of actinic keratosis, a precancerous skin condition that may become cancerous without treatment.

Sources:
1. NASA Women's Outreach Initiative, 2001.
2. National Cancer Institute, 2002.
3. National Cancer Institute, 2002.

PREVENTION & MANAGEMENT

The risk of skin cancer can be lowered with the following measures:

• Limit sun exposure, especially during the middle of the day.
• When in the sun, use a sunscreen with a sun protection factor (SPF) of at least 15.
• Wear protective clothing, sunglasses, and a hat when outdoors.
• Avoid using tanning beds or sunlamps.

Early detection of skin cancer is key to successful treatment, especially for melanoma. Examine the skin all over the body regularly for signs of new growths or changes to existing moles.

Treatment options may include:
• Surgical removal of the cancer.
• **Radiation therapy**.
• Freezing the tumor.
• **Laser therapy**.
• **Chemotherapy**.
• **Immunotherapy**.

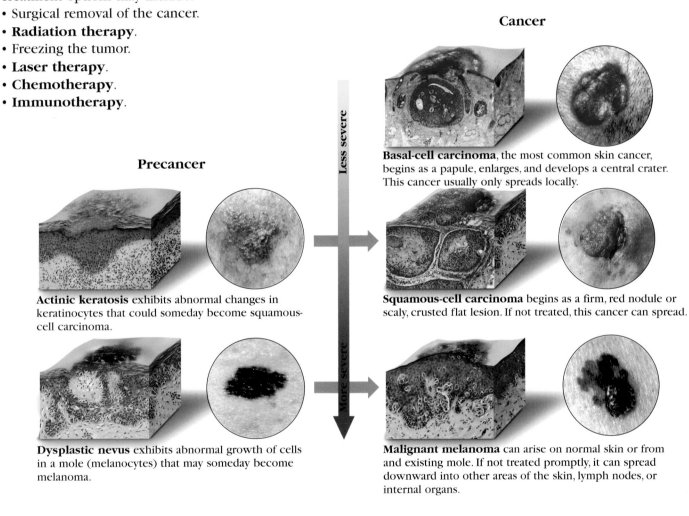

Cancer

Basal-cell carcinoma, the most common skin cancer, begins as a papule, enlarges, and develops a central crater. This cancer usually only spreads locally.

Precancer

Actinic keratosis exhibits abnormal changes in keratinocytes that could someday become squamous-cell carcinoma.

Squamous-cell carcinoma begins as a firm, red nodule or scaly, crusted flat lesion. If not treated, this cancer can spread.

Dysplastic nevus exhibits abnormal growth of cells in a mole (melanocytes) that may someday become melanoma.

Malignant melanoma can arise on normal skin or from and existing mole. If not treated promptly, it can spread downward into other areas of the skin, lymph nodes, or internal organs.

The ABCD's of Malignant Melanoma

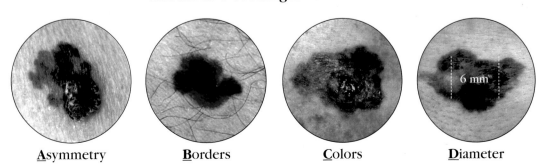

| <u>A</u>symmetry | <u>B</u>orders | <u>C</u>olors | <u>D</u>iameter |

Healthy Aging

"The old woman I shall become will be quite different from the woman I am now. Another 'I' is beginning."

George Sand
(pen name of Amandine Aurore Lucil)

The process of growing older brings with it certain changes. For women, the most significant of these is the onset of menopause. Though a time of great change, the onset of menopause can also be a time of new beginnings. Freedom from monthly periods and its associated symptoms is a refreshing change for most women. Other health issues associated with growing older can be managed through increased knowledge, staying active, and practicing preventive care. New lifestyle choices and the maintenance of healthy habits will help make the aging experience a positive one.

Topics:
    Alzheimer's Disease
    Cataracts and Macular Degeneration
    Menopause
    Osteoarthritis
    Osteoporosis

Alzheimer's disease, the most common form of **dementia**, causes a progressive loss of memory and intellectual ability.

Alzheimer's disease is the eighth leading cause of death in American adults.[1]

As more and more people live longer, the number of people affected by Alzheimer's will continue to grow.[2]

DETAILED DESCRIPTION

Alzheimer's disease (AD) slowly destroys the cells and communication pathways of the brain. Abnormalities including amyloid plaques and neurofibrillary tangles develop in the brains of those with the disease. The result is impaired memory, language deterioration, and dramatic personality changes.

RISK FACTORS

The cause of Alzheimer's disease is unknown. The major risk factors include:

- Advancing age—Alzheimer's is most common after age 65, and the risk doubles every five years after age 65.[3]
- A family history of Alzheimer's.

Other possible factors that are currently being researched include:

- Gender. Women may have a higher risk of the disease, although their higher rates may only reflect the effects of age—on average, women have longer life spans than men.
- Head injury.
- Lower levels of education.
- Genetic (inherited) factors.
- Environmental factors: scientists have found aluminum, zinc, and other metals in the brain tissue of people with AD.
- Viruses.

SYMPTOMS & SIGNS

Alzheimer's disease begins slowly and mildly, becoming more serious as the disease progresses. The average course of the disease is six to ten years and includes three stages:

- Stage 1:
  - Mild but repeated forgetfulness, especially of newly learned information.
  - Personality changes, such as becoming easily upset or anxious.
  - Disorientation in familiar surroundings.
- Stage 2:
  - Significant memory problems.
  - Depression or withdrawal.
  - Trouble with decision-making.
- Stage 3:
  - Lack of awareness of time and place.
  - Inability to recognize family and friends.
  - Suspicious or agitated demeanor.
  - Sleep disturbances.

Sources:
1. National Center for Health Statistics, 1999.
2. National Institute on Aging, 2000.
3. National Institute On Aging, 2001.

PREVENTION & MANAGEMENT

Alzheimer's disease is difficult to diagnose. Doctors first rule out other possible causes of dementia. For instance, some medications can cause Alzheimer's-like symptoms, as can health problems such as depression and alcohol abuse. A diagnosis of probable Alzheimer's can be made only after other potential causes have been eliminated. The future may bring advances in the diagnosis of Alzheimer's. Researchers are testing new brain-scanning technology that may make it easier for doctors to identify the disease.

Treatments for those suffering from Alzheimer's disease include:
• Medications, such as **cholinesterase inhibitors**, to minimize memory loss and control behavioral symptoms.
• Vitamin and mineral supplements to prevent nutrient deficiencies that can intensify symptoms.

Although there is not yet a cure for Alzheimer's disease, research is under way to explore the following treatments to manage, slow and perhaps prevent Alzheimer's disease:
• **Nonsteroidal anti-inflammatory drugs (NSAIDs)**.
• Vitamin E.
• Estrogen.
• Ginko Biloba—an extract made from the leaves of the ginko tree.
• Intellectually stimulating activities such as reading and engaging crossword puzzles or card games.

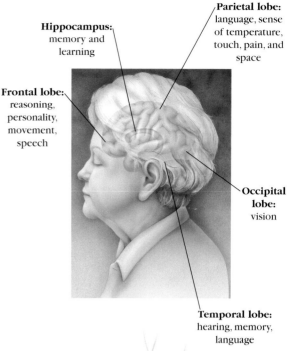

Hippocampus: memory and learning

Parietal lobe: language, sense of temperature, touch, pain, and space

Frontal lobe: reasoning, personality, movement, speech

Occipital lobe: vision

Temporal lobe: hearing, memory, language

Abnormal Cellular Structures

Granulovascular degeneration is found inside the hippocampus. An abnormally high number of fluid-filled spaces, called vacuoles, enlarge the cell's body, possibly causing the cell to malfunction or die.

Neurofibrillary tangles are bundles of filaments inside the neuron that abnormally twist around one another. Scientists believe the neurofibrillary tangles play a role in the memory loss and personality changes that the AD patient suffers.

Amyloid plaques (senile plaques) are found outside the neurons in the extracellular space of the cerebral cortex and hippocampus.

Normal neuron

Dendrites

Neurofilament

Nucleus

Vacuole

Cell body

Axon

Physical Changes in Cortex

Cerebral cortex (grey matter): thinking

Neuron cell body

Axon

White matter

Normal   **Alzheimer's**

In Alzheimer's Disease the greatest loss of neurons occurs in the cortex of the temporal and parietal lobes, causing the grey matter of that area to shrink, or atrophy.

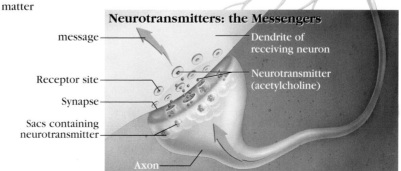

Neurotransmitters: the Messengers

message

Receptor site

Synapse

Sacs containing neurotransmitter

Dendrite of receiving neuron

Neurotransmitter (acetylcholine)

Axon

A cataract is a clouding of the eye's lens, which slowly causes vision loss. Age-related macular degeneration (AMD) is the deterioration of the part of the retina responsible for central vision, the type of eyesight that allows you do activities that require fine, sharp straight-ahead vision such as reading and driving.

Nearly half of all Americans over age 65 have cataracts.[1]

Cataracts are the leading cause of blindness in the world. But in the United States, macular degeneration is the leading cause of blindness and vision impairment in people age 60 and older.[2]

DETAILED DESCRIPTION

A cataract occurs when the protein found in the lens of the eye clumps together and clouds small areas of the eye, blocking some light from reaching the **retina** and interfering with vision.

Age-related macular degeneration (AMD) causes the **macula**, which is located near the center of the retina, to deteriorate. There are two types of AMD. Ninety percent of AMD sufferers have dry AMD. This form of AMD causes the cells in the macula to break down slowly, leading to a gradual loss of central vision.

Only 10 percent of people with AMD have wet AMD. But this type of AMD accounts for 90 percent of all blindness that is caused by the disease. In wet AMD, new blood vessels grow and leak blood and fluid under the macula, which can cause a rapid loss of central vision.

RISK FACTORS

Cataracts	AMD
• Advancing age. • Family history of cataracts. • Diabetes. • Use of corticosteroid medications. • Eye surgery. • Unprotected exposure to sunlight and light in tanning booths.	• Advancing age. • Family history of macular degeneration. • Gender—women are more likely to suffer from macular degeneration than men are. • Race—Caucasians are more likely to suffer from macular degeneration than African Americans are. • Cigarette smoking. • Elevated cholesterol.

SYMPTOMS & SIGNS

Cataracts	AMD
• Blurring of vision. • Problems with lights—for instance, seeing halos around lights or glare from headlights. • Poor night vision. • Double or multiple vision.	*Dry* • Blurred vision. • The need for increased light in order to perform tasks. • Slowly growing blind spots in the middle field of vision. *Wet* • Straight lines that appear wavy. • Rapid loss of central vision. • Blind spots.

Sources:
1. National Eye Institute, 2001.
2. National Eye Institute, 2001.

PREVENTION & MANAGEMENT

Measures that may help reduce the risk of and/or lessen the damage of cataracts and AMD include:

• Wearing sunglasses.
• Not smoking to protect against AMD.
• Eating foods rich in antioxidants, vitamins, zinc, and cartotenoids, such as leafy, green vegetables and carrots.

Regular eye exams are key to detecting cataracts and AMD. There are no treatments for dry AMD. Treatment options for cataracts and wet AMD may include:

• For cataracts: Stronger or specialized eyeglasses, such as those with magnifying lenses.
• For cataracts: Surgery in which the lens of the eye is removed and replaced with an artificial lens.
• For wet AMD: Laser surgery to slow or stop degeneration of the retina.

Normal

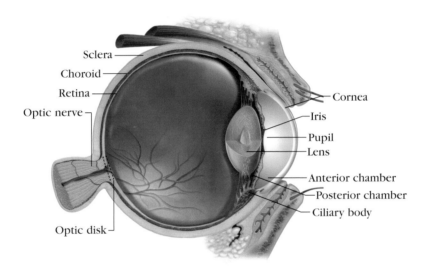

Sclera
Choroid
Retina
Optic nerve
Cornea
Iris
Pupil
Lens
Anterior chamber
Posterior chamber
Ciliary body
Optic disk

Cataract

Macular Degeneration

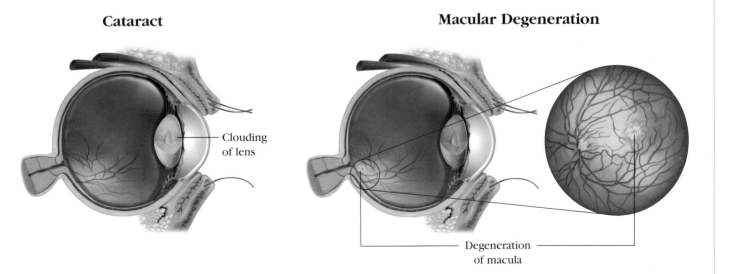

Clouding of lens

Degeneration of macula

Menopause refers to the complete cessation of a woman's menstrual cycle.

The event that marks menopause is your final menstrual period. You will know for sure that you have experienced menopause when you have not had a period in a year.[1]

Perimenopause probably begins about three to five years before your final menstrual period. It lasts until 12 months after your final period. Some signs or symptoms of menopause may appear during this time.[2]

DETAILED DESCRIPTION

Menopause is the date that marks a woman's last menstrual period. The events leading up to and following menopause are referred to as perimenopause. The perimenopausal time is associated with many physical, emotional, and mental changes. Once menopause has occurred, the ovaries produce less estrogen. This may put a woman at increased risk for several health conditions, including heart disease and osteoporosis.

SYMPTOMS & SIGNS

Physical	Emotional/Mental
• No menstrual periods. • Thinning of genital-urinary tissues, which may lead to painful intercourse. • Hot flashes, characterized by redness and/or sweating in the face, neck, and chest. • Night sweats and insomnia. • Less firm breasts. • Increased growth of facial hair. • Thinning hair on the scalp. • Thinner, less elastic skin. • Decreased muscle mass and increased fat.	• Fatigue caused by sleep deprivation. • Mood swings. • Forgetfulness. • Decreased sex drive. • Depression.

Major Health Risks

Postmenopausal women are at increased risk for the following conditions:

• Osteoporosis—bone loss is most rapid in the five to seven years after menopause.[3]
• Heart disease—leading cause of death in postmenopausal women.[4]
• Urinary incontinence—lack of estrogen can cause thinning of the urethra and bladder tissues, resulting in decreased bladder control and more frequent urge to urinate.

PREVENTION & MANAGEMENT

Menopause is a natural part of a woman's life cycle. However, this is a time when a woman can make several health-related decisions. **Hormone replacement therapy (HRT)** has been shown in some studies to reduce the risk of osteoporosis and heart disease. However, there are side effects and health risks associated with HRT use. Deciding whether to take postmenopausal hormone replacement is complicated for many women. The benefits of hormone replacement therapy (HRT) are significant, but they must be weighed against the potential risks. Women should consult with their physician about HRT to determine if it is appropriate for them.

Sources:
1. National Institute on Aging, 1999.
2. National Institute on Aging, 1999.
3. National Institutes of Heath Osteoporosis and Related Bone Diseases Resource Center, 2002.
4. National Heart, Lung, and Blood Institute, 2002.

Following is a list of the benefits and risks associated with HRT:

Benefits	Risks
• Reduced osteoporosis risk. • Reduced heart disease risk. • Reduced incontinence risk. • Decreased vaginal dryness and irritation. • Decreased hot flashes. • Increased energy.	• Increased risk of endometrial cancer (if using **ERT**). • Possible increased risk of breast cancer. • Possible increased risk of gallbladder disease. • Other potential side effects: Bloating, fluid retention, breast tenderness, headaches, mood changes, and nausea.

Whether you choose to take HRT or not, consider other options. This is a great time to re-establish a relationship with a health care provider. Your provider may encourage you to get regular **mammograms**, **colonoscopies**, and blood-work to check your **thyroid gland** and **lipid profile**. It is also important to get regular exercise and to eat a healthy diet that is high in fiber and calcium and low in fat.

25% NO SYMPTOMS
50% MINOR SYMPTOMS
25% MANY INCONVENIENT SYMPTOMS

No Symptoms

Some women experience no symptoms other than cessation of menstrual periods.

Body Changes During Menopause

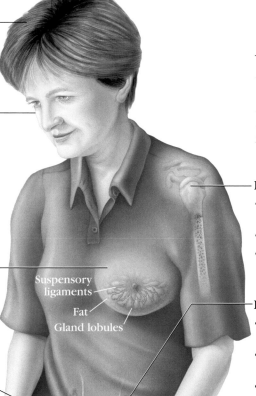

Hair Growth

• Thinning of scalp hair.

• Darkening or thickening of other body hair, such as facial hair.

Skin

• Loss of firmness, tension, and fluid.

• Decrease in melanocytes, which give skin pigment.

• Increased sensitivity to sun exposure.

Breasts

• Glandular tissue replaced with fat.

• Flattening of form.

Urinary System

• Thinning of tissues in bladder and urethra.

• Increased risk of urinary tract infections.

Suspensory ligaments
Fat
Gland lobules

Key

a = Ureter
b = Bladder
c = Urethra
d = Ovary
e = Uterus
f = Vagina

Bone

• Becomes progressively more porous and brittle.

• Increased risk of osteoporosis.

• More subject to fractures, especially the shoulder, upper arm, and hip.

Reproductive System

• Few remaining follicles (egg cells) in ovaries.

• Reproductive organs decrease in size.

• Vaginal mucosa becomes thinner, less lubricated.

• Vaginal pH changes, increasing susceptibility to infection.

• Endometriosis disappears.

96

Osteoarthritis is the thinning or destruction of cartilage in the joints.

By age 65, more than half of the U.S. population has x-ray evidence of osteoarthritis in at least one joint.[1]

Before age 45, more men than women suffer from osteoarthritis. After age 45, more women are affected.[2]

DETAILED DESCRIPTION

Osteoarthritis occurs when the joints have been damaged over time from injury or overuse. Cartilage, a protective tissue that lines the joints and helps prevent bones from rubbing together, is gradually lost, and joint pain and inflammation develop.

RISK FACTORS

A woman's risk of osteoarthritis rises with age. Other risk factors include:
• A family history of osteoarthritis.
• Excess body weight.
• History of work that involves heavy labor.
• An athletic injury.

SYMPTOMS & SIGNS

• Joint aches and pain—especially in the hips, knees, spine, and hands—during movement.
• Joint stiffness after a period of inactivity.
• Painful and knobby bone growths on the end and middle joints of the fingers.

PREVENTION & MANAGEMENT

Treatments for osteoarthritis work to reduce pain and swelling, keep joints moving safely, and avoid further damage to joints. These treatments include:
• Medicines and supplements:
    • Over-the-counter **nonsteroidal anti-inflammatory drugs**, such as aspirin, ibuprofen, and naproxen.
    • Prescription medication.
    • Oral supplements with glucosamine and chondroitin sulfate.
• Regular exercise.
• Maintaining a healthy body weight.
• Relaxation techniques.
• Surgery, if needed.

Sources:
1. National Institute of Arthritis and Musculoskeletal and Skin Diseases, 2000.
2. National Institute of Arthritis and Musculoskeletal and Skin Diseases, 2000.

Joints Affected by Osteoarthritis

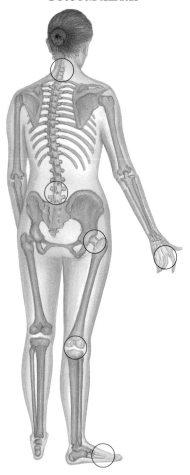

Hand and Wrist with Osteoarthritis

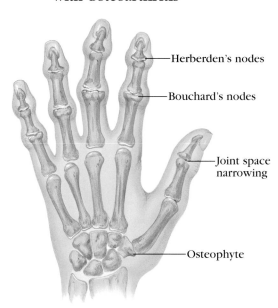

Herberden's nodes

Bouchard's nodes

Joint space narrowing

Osteophyte

Right Hip with Osteoarthritis
(anterior view)

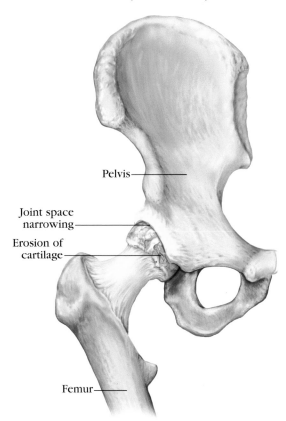

Pelvis

Joint space narrowing

Erosion of cartilage

Femur

Right Knee with Osteoarthritis
(anterior view)

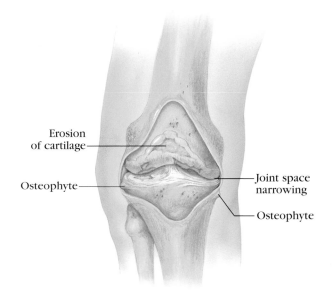

Erosion of cartilage

Osteophyte

Joint space narrowing

Osteophyte

Patella removed to visualize joint

Osteoporosis is a disease that causes bones to become thin and weak.

Women can lose up to 20 percent of their bone mass in the five to seven years after menopause, increasing their susceptibility to osteoporosis.[1]

Women are four times more likely to suffer from osteoporosis than men are.[2]

DETAILED DESCRIPTION

Osteoporosis develops when the body loses bone faster than it can make it. As a result, bones become less dense at the core and lose thickness at the surface. This increases the bones' susceptibility to fracture.

RISK FACTORS

Women have a higher risk of osteoporosis than men do. In addition to gender, risk factors include:
• Advancing age or postmenopausal status.
• An inactive lifestyle.
• A small bone structure.
• Low intake of calcium.
• Smoking.
• Excess alcohol consumption.
• Certain medications, such as glucocorticoids (which are used to control diseases such as arthritis and asthma), some anti-seizure drugs, certain sleeping pills, some hormones used to treat endometriosis, and some cancer drugs.
• Excessive thyroid hormone in the body.
• Race—Caucasian and Asian women have a higher risk of developing osteoporosis.
• Breastfeeding. *Note:* women who lose bone mineral during lactation recover bone density within 6 months.

SYMPTOMS & SIGNS

Osteoporosis is often called a silent disease because it causes no symptoms until bones become very weak. At that point symptoms may include:
• Low back pain.
• Loss of height over time, accompanied by a stooped posture.
• Fractures that occur after a fall or a non-major injury.

PREVENTION & MANAGEMENT

Osteoporosis is usually preventable. Protective steps include:
• Good eating and exercise habits, ideally from early in life. Building strong bones at a young age will lessen the effect of the natural bone loss that begins to occur around age 30.
• Adequate intake of calcium (1,000 mg if premenopausal/1,500 mg if postmenopausal) and vitamin D.
• Regular exercise, including weight-bearing activities, which put stress on the bones.
• Not smoking.
• Limited alcohol consumption.
• Consulting with a physician to find out if you should have a bone mineral density test.

Sources:
1. NIH Osteoporosis and Related Bone Diseases Resource Center, 2002.
2. National Institutes of Health, 2002.

Drug therapy can be used to prevent and to treat osteoporosis. The following drugs have been approved by the FDA to preserve or increase bone masses and maintain bone quality to reduce the risk of fractures:

- **Estrogen Replacement Therapy (ERT)**.
- **Hormone Replacement Therapy (HRT)**.
- Biophosphonates (a class of drugs that slows down bone loss).
- Selective estrogen receptor modulators (SERMs) that has many estrogen-like properties, but does not slow down bone loss as much as estrogen.
- Hormones to regulate calcium and bone metabolism.

Other methods to prevent and treat osteoporosis are currently being researched and studied. Women should consult with their doctor to determine the best plan of treatment.

Joints Affected by Osteoporosis

What is Osteoporosis

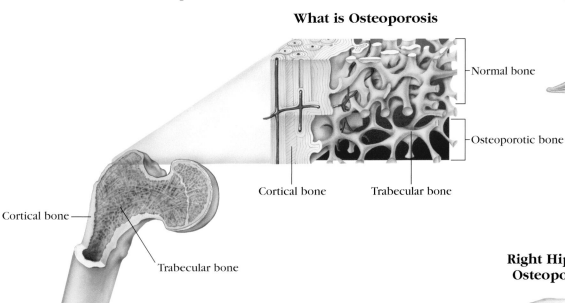

Normal bone

Osteoporotic bone

Cortical bone

Trabecular bone

Cortical bone

Trabecular bone

Femur

Right Hip with Osteoporosis

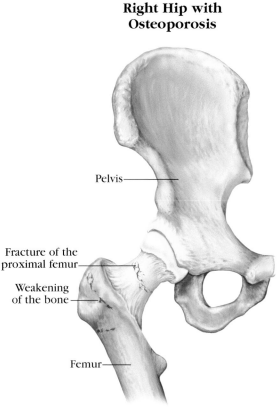

Pelvis

Fracture of the proximal femur

Weakening of the bone

Femur

Postmenopausal Osteoporosis

This type of osteoporosis usually occurs in women several years after menopause. At this time, women's ovaries produce less estrogen. In the absence of estrogen, bone resorption increases, dropping overall bone mass below the maintenance density level and risking fracture.

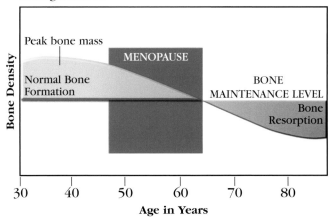

Peak bone mass

MENOPAUSE

Normal Bone Formation

BONE MAINTENANCE LEVEL

Bone Resorption

Bone Density

30   40   50   60   70   80

Age in Years

Emotional Wellness

"Our feelings are our most genuine path to knowledge."
Audre Lorde

Emotional wellness is an essential ingredient of good health. Women often face different challenges than men in achieving emotional health. Women are twice as likely to develop depression and experience higher rates of some anxiety disorders than men do. Scientists are only now beginning to discover the effects of biological and psychosocial factors on mental health and mental illness in both women and men. More often than not, a woman's emotional health suffers as she tries to balance the competing demands of family, marriage, and career. A woman's emotional needs are as important as her physical ones, and the two often affect one another. Fortunately, many new treatment options exist for dealing with mood and anxiety disorders, whether mild or more severe.

Topics:
    Generalized Anxiety, Panic and Post-Traumatic Stress Disorders
    Depression
    Postpartum Depression

In addition, researchers are currently studying the special problems of treatment for serious mental illness during pregnancy and the postpartum period. Research on women's health has grown substantially in the last 20 years. Today's studies are helping to clarify the risk and protective factors for mental disorders in women and to improve women's mental health treatment outcome.

Anxiety disorders are a group of serious medical illnesses that involve excessive, irrational fear and dread.

Generalized anxiety disorder affects about 4 million adult Americans and about twice as many women as men.[1]

DETAILED DESCRIPTION

Anxiety disorders affect approximately 19 million American adults.[2] These disorders include generalized anxiety, panic, obsessive-compulsive, social anxiety, and specific phobias. This chapter focuses on the disorders that are more prevalent in women than in men.[3]

Generalized anxiety disorder (GAD) is an illness characterized by excessive worry and tension. GAD sufferers regularly anticipate disaster and cannot seem to shake their concerns, although most realize the intensity of the worry is unwarranted.

Episodes of *panic disorder* involve feelings of intense fear that come on suddenly and repeatedly without warning. Because of the unpredictability of the episodes, people with panic disorder may avoid all situations that they associate with panic attacks.

Post-traumatic stress disorder (PTSD) is a debilitating condition that can develop following a terrifying event. This event may have been a direct life threat to the sufferer or someone close to the sufferer, or the triggering event could have been witnessed, such as massive death and destruction. PTSD sufferers may have persistent frightening thoughts and memories called flashbacks throughout the day and night. PTSD is diagnosed only if the symptoms last more than a month, but the illness can last indefinitely.

RISK FACTORS

Generalized Anxiety Disorder (GAD)	Panic Disorder	Post-Traumatic Stress Disorder (PTSD)
• Gender: Affects about twice as many women as men. • Age: Risk is highest between childhood and middle age. • Genetic vulnerability. • Environmental influences.	• Gender: Twice as common in women as in men. • Age: Most often begins during late adolescence or early adulthood. • Genetic vulnerability. • Environmental influences.	• Experiencing or witnessing a traumatic event. • Gender: Women are more likely to develop PTSD than men are. • Genetic vulnerability. • Environmental influences.

SYMPTOMS & SIGNS

Generalized Anxiety Disorder (GAD)	Panic Disorder	Post-Traumatic Stress Disorder (PTSD)
• Feeling anxious or worried most of the time, often for no reason, for at least six months. • Difficulty relaxing and falling asleep. • Muscle tension, fatigue, sweating, trembling, twitching, hot flashes. • Feeling light-headed or out of breath. • Nausea. • Frequent need to urinate. • Becoming startled easily. • Difficulty concentrating.	• Increased heart rate. • Feeling sweaty, weak, faint, flushed, chilled, or dizzy. • Tingling or numb hands. • Nausea. • Chest pains or smothering sensations. • Fear of impending doom or loss of control. • Feelings of going crazy, losing control, or being on the verge of death. Note: Attack may peak within 10 minutes, but some symptoms may last longer.	• Experiencing terrifying recollections during the day or night. • Sleeping problems. • Feeling detached or numb. • Difficulty being affectionate. • Feeling irritable, aggressive, or even violent. • Losing interest in previously enjoyable activities. • Becoming startled easily. • Extreme distress at reminders of the traumatic event. Symptoms seem to be worse if the triggering event was deliberately initiated by a person, such as rape or kidnapping, as opposed to a natural disaster.

PREVENTION & MANAGEMENT

Although there are no established methods of preventing the onset of anxiety disorders, the ultimate goal of mental health research is to find ways to prevent these illnesses. It is important however, to consult with your doctor if you experience symptoms of anxiety so it can be determined if they are due to an anxiety disorder, some other medical condition, or both.

Options in the treatment and management of anxiety disorders include:

- Cognitive-behavioral therapy— Therapy targeted at changing negative, self-defeating thought patterns and behaviors.
- Antidepressant medication.
- Antianxiety medication.
- Aerobic exercise.
- Relaxation techniques, including yoga and breathing exercises.
- Well-balanced diet.
- Support groups.
- Outreach to family and friends.
- Adequate sleep.

An anxiety disorder is often accompanied by another type of anxiety disorder, depression, or substance abuse, which should be treated along with the disorder.

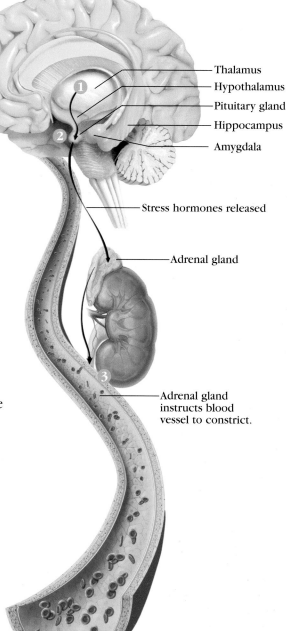

Thalamus
Hypothalamus
Pituitary gland
Hippocampus
Amygdala

Stress hormones released

Adrenal gland

Adrenal gland instructs blood vessel to constrict.

Flight or Fight Response

Several parts of the brain play an important role in fear and anxiety disorders. In particular, the amygdala and hippocampus control the body's "fight or flight" response to stress.

1. When a threatening event is perceived, these centers activate the hypothalamic-pituitary-adrenocortical (HPA) axis.

2. Once activated, the HPA axis alerts the sympathetic nervous system…

3. Which releases stress hormones. In people with anxiety, the HPA axis is thought to be hyperactive, triggering the body's stress response when no external threat is present.

Sources:
1. National Institute of Mental Health, 2002.
2. National Institute of Mental Health, 2002.
3. National Institute of Mental Health, 2002.

Depression is a mood disorder that affects the mind and body.

Before adolescence, boys and girls experience equal rates of depression. By high school, females are twice as likely as males to have experienced a depressive episode.[1]

Depression rates are highest in women who are unhappily married, followed by women who are divorced or separated.[2]

DETAILED DESCRIPTION

Depression affects more than 19 million Americans each year. Twice as many women as men experience depression.[3] Researchers are investigating the unique biological, psychosocial, and environmental factors that may be associated with higher rates of depression among women.[4] Genetics, sex hormones, reactions to life stress and trauma, cognitive style, and interpersonal relationships may all contribute to the increased prevalence in women.

Depression is associated with a chemical imbalance in the brain. Neurotransmitters are chemicals that carry messages among **neurons** that affect behavior, mood, and thought. Two of the neurotransmitters that play a role in depression are norepinephrine and serotonin. Norepinephrine and serotonin's activity are low when a person is depressed.

RISK FACTORS

- Family history of depression.
- Hormonal changes, such as during the premenstrual period or after childbirth. *(Note: Refer to the "Premenstrual Syndrome" and "Postpartum Depression" chapters for further discussion.)*
- Environmental stressors and psychosocial factors, such as difficult relationships, financial problems, major life changes, pessimism, low self-esteem, or insufficient social support.
- History of sexual or physical abuse.

SYMPTOMS & SIGNS

Not all feelings of sadness indicate depression; in fact, it is normal to experience some symptoms of depression after a traumatic life event without being clinically depressed. Depression is diagnosed when three or more of the following symptoms persist for two weeks or longer:
- Persistent sad, anxious, or "empty" mood.
- Loss of interest in usually pleasurable activities.
- Restlessness, irritability, or excessive crying.
- Feelings of guilt, worthlessness, helplessness, or hopelessness.
- Sleeping too much or too little.
- Appetite and/or weight changes.
- Decreased energy (fatigue).
- Thoughts of death or suicide, or suicide attempts.
- Difficulty concentrating, remembering, or making decisions.
- Persistent physical symptoms that do not respond to treatment, such as headaches, digestive disorders, and chronic pain.

PREVENTION & MANAGEMENT

Preventing depression is an important but challenging endeavor as it requires a timely diagnostic evaluation of risk factors and any symptoms or signs. Consult with your doctor and/or mental health professional to see if you are at risk for depression and to determine appropriate preventive measures.

Options in the treatment and management of depression include:

- Psychotherapy:
  - Cognitive-behavioral therapy—Therapy targeted at changing negative, self-defeating thought patterns and behaviors.
  - Interpersonal therapy—Therapy that focuses on interpersonal relationships and improving communication skills.
  - Psychodynamic therapy—Therapy that helps the patient explore how past experiences influence current perceptions and behaviors.
- Antidepressant medications. There are several types of antidepressants. A physician can help the patient find the most effective medication.
- Regular exercise.
- Diet rich in omega-3 essential fatty acids (found in fish and fish oil), calcium, and folic acid.
- Support groups.

If you think you may have depression, the National Institute of Mental Health has a helpful booklet, "Stories of Depression: Does This Sound Like You?" which you can find online at…
http://www.nimh.nih.gov/publicat/stories depression.pdf

The Role of Neurotransmitters

Neurotransmitters are chemical messengers that carry messages among neurons that affect behavior, mood, and thought. Two of the neurotransmitters that play a role in depression are norepinephrine and serotonin.

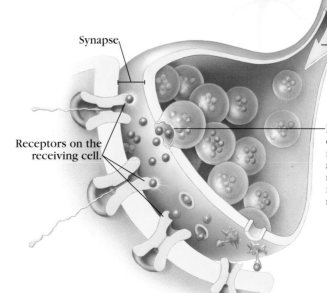

The message is passed to the end of the axon.

In the axon, sacs containing norepinephrine and serotonin are stimulated to release into the synapse.

Synapse

Receptors on the receiving cell.

Serotonin and norepinephrine cross the synapse to bind to their receptors on the receiving cell.

Neurotransmitter Activity in Depression

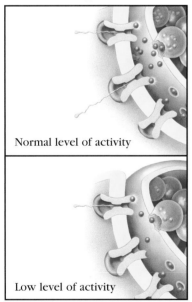

Normal level of activity

Low level of activity

Depression is associated with a chemical imbalance in the brain. Norepinephrine and serotonin's activity are low when a person is depressed.

Sources:
1. National Institute of Mental Health, 2000.
2. National Institute of Mental Health, 2000.
3. National Institute of Mental Health, 2000.
4. American Psychological Association Summit on Women and Depression, 2002.

Postpartum depression is a psychiatric disorder associated with pregnancy and childbirth that affects about 10 percent of new mothers in the United States.[1]

At least 33 percent of women who have had postpartum depression have a recurrence of symptoms after giving birth to their next child.[2]

About 50 percent of women experience the "baby blues," with crying spells and mood swings, after giving birth.[3]

DETAILED DESCRIPTION

After childbirth, a combination of biological changes and environmental stresses may trigger symptoms of depression or symptoms that are similar to depression. Beginning a few days after delivery, it is normal for a new mother to experience the "baby blues," a state of heightened emotional reactivity characterized by crying spells and mood swings. These feelings subside in a matter of days or weeks. Some new mothers, however, experience intense feelings of sadness, despair, anxiety, and irritability that disrupt their ability to function. This is known as postpartum depression.[4]

RISK FACTORS

Risk factors associated with postpartum depression include:
- Previous postpartum depression.
- Personal history of depression.
- Personal history of severe premenstrual syndrome (PMS).
- Lack of social support.
- Medical illnesses such as **thyroid** deficiency, which can occur as a result of childbirth and mimics the symptoms of depression.

SYMPTOMS & SIGNS

"Baby Blues"	Postpartum Depression
• Symptoms appear three to five days after delivery and subside within two weeks. • Episodes of crying with little provocation. • Mood swings.	• Symptoms arise within four weeks after the birth. • Feelings of doubt, guilt, hopelessness, or helplessness. • Trouble completing tasks, like caring for the baby. • Appetite changes. • Loss of pleasure in normal activities. • Excessive concern about the baby, or lack of interest in the baby. • Thoughts of harming the baby or oneself. • Difficulty sleeping, even when the baby is asleep. • Symptoms persist for weeks or months and interfere with daily functioning.

Sources:
1. National Institute of Mental Health, 2000.
2. Office on Women's Health, 2001.
3. Miller LJ (ed): *Postpartum Mood Disorder.* Washington, DC: American Psychiatric Press, 1999, p. 4. <www.appi.org>
4. Office on Women's Health, 2001.

PREVENTION & MANAGEMENT

Choices that may play a preventive role in the development of postpartum depression include:

• Rest—for instance, try to nap when the baby naps.
• Talk about your feelings to a supportive person.
• Reach out to family and friends for support and help.
• Make it a point to get out of the house each day.

If you experience the symptoms of postpartum depression, it is important to tell your doctor. Treatment options include:

• **Psychotherapy.** May include learning coping skills and techniques to reduce stress, facilitate adjustment to new roles and improve interpersonal support.
• Antidepressant medication. Different antidepressants can affect breastfeeding infants differently, with some more likely to cause side effects than others. Breastfeeding mothers should consult their doctors to determine the most suitable option.
• Support groups.

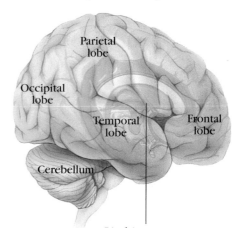

The Brain
(Lateral View)

Parietal lobe

Occipital lobe

Temporal lobe

Frontal lobe

Cerebellum

Limbic system seen deep within the brain. This system of neural structures is involved in emotional behavior.

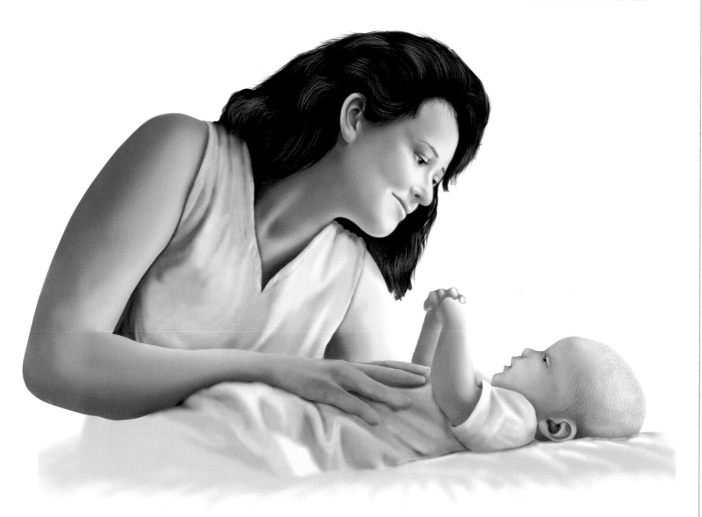

Healthy Lifestyles

*"You don't get to choose how you're going to die. Or when.
You can decide how you're going to live—now."*

Joan Baez

Tips for a healthy life include:

- Exercise regularly: 30 minutes of regular exercise on most, if not all days.
- Eat a low fat, low-cholesterol, high fiber diet with at least 5 servings of fruits and vegetables a day.
- Maintain a healthy body weight.
- Limit alcohol consumption to one drink per day.
- Don't smoke or use illegal drugs.
- Get 6 to 8 hours of sleep a night.
- Limit sun exposure and don't use artificial tanning beds.
- Practice safe sex.
- Get yearly pap smears.
- Practice regular breast self-exams, and if over age 40, annual mammograms.
- Learn which diseases and conditions you have a family history of and share with your health professional.
- Stay connected with family and friends.
- Consult a licensed health care provider if you have any health care concerns or questions.

(Sources: Centers for Disease Control, 2002, National Women's Health Information Center, 2000)

Topics:

Physical Activity

Dangers of Excess Weight

Diet and Nutrition

Dangers of Alcohol

Dangers of Smoking

Regular physical activity enhances a woman's overall health.

Almost 70 percent of American women aged 25 – 64 do not engage in regular leisure-time physical activity.[1]

As with other age groups, physically active postmenopausal women tend to have greater bone density than sedentary postmenopausal women, thus making them less at risk for osteoporosis.[2]

DETAILED DESCRIPTION

Physical inactivity is more common in women than in men. The U.S. Surgeon General recommends that women engage in at least 30 minutes of brisk physical activity (such as walking) most, if not all days a week.

There are three types of physical activity: aerobic exercise, strength training, and stretching. Aerobic exercise improves cardiovascular health by working the heart and lungs. An additional benefit to aerobic exercise is that it usually uses the weight of the body against the forces of gravity as resistance, which helps preserve bone density. Strength training, which typically utilizes hand or machine weights, improves motor strength and power, muscle tone, coordination, and balance. Strength training should always be balanced and include strengthening both the flexing and the extending (opposing) muscles. Stretching keeps the body flexible, allows the muscles used in aerobic and strength training to recover, and helps prevent injury.

The health benefits associated with physical activity include:
- Healthy weight management.
- Improved mental health.
- Lower heart disease risk.
- Lower blood pressure.
- Improved cholesterol.
- Lower risk of diabetes.
- Lower risk of osteoporosis.
- Increased energy level.
- Better-quality sleep and greater ease falling asleep.

RISK FACTORS

The benefits associated with physical activity far outweigh the risks; however, it is important to take care when starting a new exercise regimen. Women over the age of 50 or those with a chronic health condition, such as heart disease, diabetes, or asthma should consult with their health care provider before beginning any exercise program.

PREVENTION & MANAGEMENT

Engaging in any amount of physical activity will have a protective effect on health. Start with short periods of activity, then gradually do the activity more often and for longer periods of time.

When exercising aerobically, it is important to monitor your heart rate. The following chart lists healthy target heart rate zones for exercise, according to age. To determine your exercising heart rate per minute, locate your pulse on your wrist or neck. Count the number of pulses for ten seconds and multiply by six. Your exercising heart rate should fall within the range listed for your age.

Healthy Heart Rate Target Zones by Age[3]

Age	Target Heart Rate Zone
20 years	100–150 beats per minute
25 years	98–146 beats per minute
30 years	95–142 beats per minute
35 years	93–138 beats per minute
40 years	90–135 beats per minute
45 years	88–131 beats per minute
50 years	85–127 beats per minute
55 years	83–123 beats per minute
60 years	80–120 beats per minute
65 years	78–116 beats per minute
70 years	75–113 beats per minute

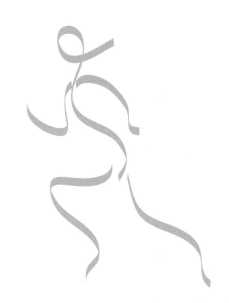

Activity	Calories Burned per Hour*
Running, 10 mph	1280
Jogging, 6 mph	654
Walking, 4½ mph	440
Walking, 2 mph	198

*These figures are for a person who weighs 150 pounds (68 kg)
mph = miles per hour
yds. = yards
min. = minute

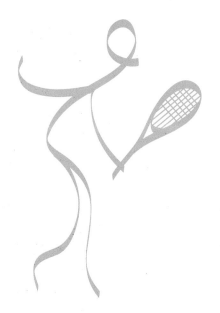

Activity	Calories Burned per Hour*
Racquetball	588
Tennis, singles	450
Tennis, doubles	312
Golf (2-some, carrying clubs)	324

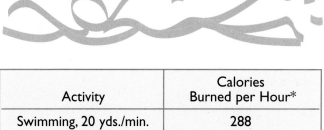

Activity	Calories Burned per Hour*
Swimming, 20 yds./min.	288
Swimming, 45 yds./min.	522
Bicycling, 5 mph	174
Bicycling, 13 mph	612

Sources:
1. National Health Interview Survey, 2001.
2. Osteoporosis and Related Bone Diseases Resource Center, 2001.
3. National Heart, Lung, and Blood Institute, 2002.

A woman is considered overweight if her weight is higher than the ideal range for her height. Many health risks are associated with being overweight.

Half of all adult American women are overweight.[1]

More than 60 percent of African American, Mexican American, and Native American women are overweight or obese. Asian American women, in general, have the lowest rates of obesity.[2]

DETAILED DESCRIPTION

Maintaining a healthy body weight throughout life is an important part of healthy aging. Significant weight gain during adulthood is associated with higher rates of chronic disease and greater likelihood of premature death.

RISK FACTORS

Risk factors for excess weight include:
- Genetics—Inherited factors include metabolism and where fat is distributed on the body.
- Little or no physical activity.
- Caloric intake that exceeds daily **calorie** needs.
- Hormone imbalance.

SYMPTOMS & SIGNS

A healthy body weight range is determined by dividing your weight, measured in kilograms, by the square of your height, measured in meters. This is known as your body mass index (BMI). To calculate your BMI:
1. Convert weight in pounds to kilograms by dividing by 2.2.
2. Convert height in inches to meters by multiplying by 0.0254.
3. Square height by multiplying it times itself.
4. Divide weight in kilograms (#1) by height in meters squared (#3).

	Healthy	Overweight	Obese
BMI	18.5-24.9	25-29.9	30+

The way that excess fat is distributed on the body plays an important role in the health risks associated with it:
- Apple-shaped figure:
  - Excess fat is distributed around the abdomen.
  - Common in postmenopausal women.
  - Associated with increased overall health risk.
- Pear-shaped figure:
  - Excess fat is distributed around the hips and buttocks.
  - More common in women.
  - Associated with increased risk of osteoarthritis.

As the amount of excess body fat increases—especially if distributed around the abdomen—so does the risk of:
- Cardiovascular disease.
- Type 2 diabetes.
- Some forms of cancer, especially breast, colon, and endometrial.
- **Pulmonary embolism**.
- Gallbladder disease.
- **Obstructive sleep apnea**.
- Osteoarthritis.
- Irregular menstrual cycles and infertility. Abdominal obesity is linked to **polycystic ovary syndrome (PCOS)**, a cause of infertility in women.
- Complications during surgery.

PREVENTION & MANAGEMENT

To maintain a healthy body weight, limit daily caloric intake through reasonable serving sizes, consume foods low in fat and refined sugars, and engage in regular physical activity. A woman's caloric needs are determined by the amount of muscle present and by her level of physical activity.

A general formula for calculating daily calories needed for a target body weight is:

1. Convert weight from pounds to kilograms by dividing by 2.2.
2. Multiply weight in kilograms by 25. The number you get equals your daily calorie needs in order to maintain the target body weight.

Tips for physical activity include making exercise a part of your normal routine. Here are some examples:

• Walk at least 10 to 20 minutes daily.
• Take the stairs instead of the elevator.
• Join a sports team or dance class.
• Work outdoors in the garden.

For a more in-depth discussion on physical activity, please refer to the "Physical Activity" chapter.

If you are overweight or obese, talk with your doctor about the best weight loss plan for you.

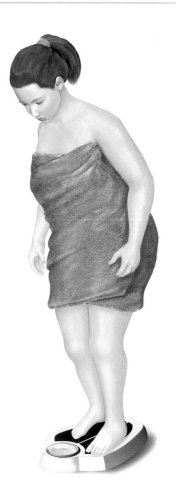

Excess Fat Distribution

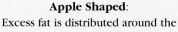

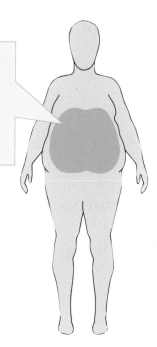

Apple Shaped:
Excess fat is distributed around the abdomen. Common in men, postmenopausal women, and with aging. Associated with increased risk of Type 2 diabetes.

Pear Shaped:
Excess fat is distributed around the hips and buttocks. Common in women. Associated with increased risk of osteoarthritis.

Sources:
1. National Institute of Diabetes and Digestive and Kidney Diseases, 2000.
2. National Institute of Diabetes and Digestive and Kidney Diseases, 2000.

Good eating habits can improve health and reduce the risk of chronic disease.

Women should consume 25 to 30 grams of fiber each day.[1]

For women, the recommended daily allowance (RDA) for iron is 15 milligrams per day, 5 more milligrams than the RDA for men.[2]

DETAILED DESCRIPTION

Healthy diet and good nutrition habits provide an array of health benefits throughout life. Eating foods that are low in cholesterol, saturated fats, and trans-fatty acids and high in fiber and whole grains helps protect the body against heart disease. In addition, fruits, vegetables and other plant-based foods like whole grains and legumes offer protective effects against cancer and other diseases. Eating such foods and engaging in physical activity further help prevent obesity thereby reducing a woman's risk for cancer, heart disease, and diabetes.

Diet

Healthy diet and nutrition habits involve eating a balanced variety of foods, from the following food categories:

- *Carbohydrates*—Should account for 55 percent of daily calories. Carbohydrates supply the body with energy. Plant foods high in starch are called complex carbohydrates. These are excellent sources of energy because they are often fat-free and carry valuable vitamins, minerals and fiber with them. Legumes, vegetables, fruits, cereals, rice, pasta, bread, nuts and seeds are all good sources of carbohydrates.

- *Fats and oils*—Should account for 30 percent or less of daily calorie intake. Fats and oils are essential to a healthy diet, contributing energy and providing fat-soluble vitamins such as A, D, and E. All dietary fats contain varying amounts of saturated and unsaturated fatty acids. Saturated fat intake should be limited to less than 10 percent of calories, or less than 7 percent if blood cholesterol levels are high. Excess consumption of saturated fats can contribute to heart disease. Most sources of saturated fat are animal foods such as high-fat meats, whole milk, and other full-fat dairy products such as butter and cream. A few plant foods, such as palm kernel oil and coconut oil, are also high in saturated fat. Unsaturated fats help sustain normal growth and can help lower blood cholesterol and triglyceride levels. Good sources of unsaturated fat are plant oils from corn, safflower seeds and soybeans, as well as olive oil or canola oil. Liquid oils are preferred over hydrogenated fats, because the latter contribute trans-fatty acids that, like saturated fats, can raise blood cholesterol. Fish (such as salmon, tuna and mackerel) and fish oil contribute omega-3 fatty acids that can help to lower triglyceride levels. Plant stanols and sterols, which are available in margarine form, may help lower blood LDL cholesterol.

- *Protein*—Should account for about 15 percent of daily calorie intake. Proteins provide the structural core of the body and maintain many bodily functions and organs. Proteins are made of amino acids. Of 22 total, there are nine essential amino acids that the body can get only from dietary protein. Meat, fish, eggs, and dairy products are significant sources of protein that contain all nine amino acids, but legumes, including soy and other beans, in combination with other plant-based foods or fat free dairy products, can supply complete proteins as well.

Supplements

Vitamins and minerals are needed to convert food to energy, create amino and fatty acids, generate tissue growth, and drive many other internal processes. Although a varied and nutritious diet will usually meet a woman's recommended daily allowances for vitamins and minerals, taking a supplement may offer additional protection against disease.

Following is a list of six essential vitamins and minerals and the amounts of them that women need every day.
- Vitamin A: 800 mcg **RE (Retinol Equivalents)**
- Vitamin B-12: 2.4 mcg
- Vitamin D: 5 mcg
- Calcium: 1,000 mg if premenopausal/1,500 mg if postmenopausal. Pregnant and breastfeeding women require 1200-1500 mg per day.
- Iron: 15 mg (30 mg if pregnant)
- Zinc: 12 mg (15 mg if pregnant)

Although they often do not get adequate amounts of calcium and vitamin D (both of which play a vital role in preventing osteoporosis), it is essential for women of all ages to get their daily required doses, often with the help of a supplement.

Likewise, women may not get enough dietary folate (folic acid) found in fortified flour, supplemented cereals, enhanced orange juice, and legumes like lentils. Women need 180 mcg of dietary folate daily, but more during pregnancy (400 mcg).

SYMPTOMS & SIGNS

Health risks associated with an unhealthy diet and/or poor nutrition include:
- Anemia.
- Anorexia.
- Osteoporosis.
- Obesity.
- Underweight.
- Depression.
- Impaired immune system.
- Aggravated premenstrual syndrome (PMS).
- Type 2 diabetes.
- High blood pressure.
- Heart disease.
- Cancer.
- Liver disease.
- Alcoholism.

Vitamin A
* RDA: 800 mcg RE
- Night vision
- Growth and tissue healing

Vegetarian Sources:
Beta-carotene in yellow, orange and dark green leafy vegetables is converted to vitamin A in the body
Animal sources:
Cheese, eggs, chicken, liver

Vitamin B-12
* RDA: 2.4 mcg
- DNA metabolism
- Red blood cell formation
- Central nervous system maintenance

Vegetarian Sources:
Fortified cereals
Fermented Miso
Animal sources:
Milk, eggs, yogurt, fish, crab, oysters, liver, kidney, muscle meats

Vitamin D
* RDA: 5 mcg/day
- Maintenance of bones and teeth

Vegetarian Sources:
Sunlight
(30 minutes per week mild exposure)
Animal sources:
Vitamin D-fortified milk, fish-liver oil, egg yolks, butter, liver

Calcium
* RDA: 1,000 mg
- Maintenance of bones and teeth

Vegetarian Sources:
Broccoli, kale, collard greens, mustard greens, spinach
Animal sources:
Milk, yogurt, cheese, ice cream, sardines, salmon

Iron
* RDA: 15 mg
- Formation of hemoglobin, which red blood cells use to carry oxygen to all cells in the body

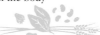

Vegetarian Sources:
Dried beans, nuts, spinach, whole grains, strawberries
Animal sources:
Beef, liver, chicken, tuna, shrimp

Zinc
* RDA: 12 mg
- Protein synthesis, DNA replication
- Many enzyme reactions

Vegetarian Sources:
Legumes, seeds, nuts
Animal sources:
Meat, poultry, oysters, eggs, milk products

Remember:
A good diet should go hand in hand with the right amount of physical activity. For more information please refer to the physical activity chapter.

USDA Food Guide Pyramid

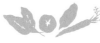

Fats, Oils and Sweets
use sparingly

Milk, Yogurt and Cheese
2-3 Servings

Meat, Poultry, Fish, Dry Beans, Eggs and Nuts
2-3 Servings

Vegetable
3-5 Servings

Fruit
2-4 Servings

Bread, Cereal, Rice and Pasta
6-11 Servings

Sources:
1. National Cancer Institute, 2001.
2. National Women's Health Information Center, 1998.

The health benefits associated with moderate alcohol consumption include reduced heart disease risk and higher HDL ("good") cholesterol levels. Excessive alcohol consumption, however, can lead to numerous health problems.

In a survey, 28.6 percent of women aged 18–25 admitted to an episode of binge drinking, in which they consumed five or more drinks on a single occasion at least once in the 30 days prior to the survey. 11.5 percent of women aged 26 and over admitted to binge drinking.[1]

As compared to men, the long-term effects of chronic alcohol abuse take a heavier toll on women's bodies and progress more rapidly.[2]

DETAILED DESCRIPTION

Moderate alcohol consumption, one drink per day, may offer health benefits, but with greater alcohol use, the risk for heart disease and other health problems begins to increase. A standard drink is generally considered to be 12 ounces of beer, 5 ounces of wine, or 1.5 ounces of 80-proof distilled spirits.

Alcohol affects women differently than men. Women become more impaired than men do after drinking the same amount of alcohol, even after differences in body weight are taken into account.

RISK FACTORS

Women with one or more of the following conditions are advised not to consume alcohol:
- Family history of alcoholism.
- Pregnancy.
- High **triglyceride** levels.
- Liver disease.
- Personal history of heart failure.
- Uncontrolled high blood pressure.
- Use of certain medications: check label and with your health care provider for restrictions.

SYMPTOMS & SIGNS

The long-term consequences of chronic alcohol abuse affect every system in the body. Symptoms vary according to the length and degree of alcohol abuse and may include the following:
- Liver:
  - Fatty liver disease.
  - Alcohol-induced hepatitis.
  - Cirrhosis, in which liver cells die and scar irreversibly.
- Nervous System:
  - Persistent short-term memory loss.
  - Chronic double vision and problems with balance.
  - Pain or loss of sensation in the arms and legs.
  - Loss of intelligence.
- Cardiovascular System:
  - High blood pressure.
  - Faster development of ateriosclerosis (hardening of the arteries).
- Digestive System:
  - Irritation of the stomach lining.
  - Ulcers.
  - **Pancreatitis**.
  - Ruptured veins in the esophagus.
  - Cancer of the esophagus, stomach, and liver.

Sources:
1. National Household Survey on Drug Abuse, 2000.
2. National Institute on Alcohol and Alcoholism, 2001.

- Reproductive System:
  - Menstrual disorders: painful menstruation, heavy flow, premenstrual discomfort, and irregular or absent cycles. May also lead to early menopause.
  - Disruptions in **ovulation**.
  - Damage to developing fetus in pregnant women.

Chronic alcohol abusers who suddenly stop drinking may experience severe withdrawal symptoms, including shaking, anxiety, hallucinations, and seizures.

PREVENTION & MANAGEMENT

If you do not already drink, don't start. If you do, limit consumption to one drink per day. Problems with alcohol abuse should be brought to the attention of a medical professional, who can recommend ways to get help.

Cardiovascular System

Chronic alcohol use can cause serious damage such as elevating your blood pressure, hastening arteriosclerosis and causing cardiomyopathy, a damaged and weakened heart muscle. In some people, however, heart disease can result from even moderate drinking.

Dilated left ventricle of heart (cardiomyopathy)

Nervous System

Alcohol can damage the brain and nerves. Excessive intake of alcohol can leave a person with temporary memory loss (blackouts) or lead to a loss of consciousness, or coma.

Neuron

Liver

The liver is frequently effected in chronic alcohol abuse. Consequences can include fatty liver disease (an accumulation of fat droplets inside liver cells) alcohol-induced hepatitis and cirrhosis.

Cirrhosis

Hepatic sinusoid in liver tissue

Liver cells

Alcohol passing into liver cell

Alcohol passing through sinusoid wall

Excess alcohol continues to circulate

Alcohol Absorption

Alcohol, absorbed through the walls of the stomach and small intestine, is carried by the blood vessels to the liver to be metabolized. Here, alcohol in the blood flows through the sinusoids and sinusoid walls and enters liver cells.

Esophageal cancer

Esophageal varices

Normal liver cell

Lipid droplets increased

Liver cell in fatty liver disease

Stomach wall absorbing alcohol

Gastritis

Gastric ulcer

Reproduction

Alcohol can cause serious problems for an unborn baby that can affect its entire life. Alcohol can also be passed along to a baby through breast milk.

Duodenal ulcer

Stomach cancer

Pancreatitis

Digestive System

Alcohol can damage many of the organs of the digestive system. Occurring frequently in alcoholics with cirrhosis, esophageal varices (dilated veins in the esophagus) may rupture and hemorrhage.

Maternal blood

Alcohol passing through placental barrier

Fetal blood vessels

118

Smoking causes a variety of chronic conditions and serious diseases, and plays a major role in the mortality of U.S. women.

Among continuing smokers, a woman's annual risk for death more than doubles as compared with persons who have never smoked in all age groups from 45 through 74 years.[1]

Cigarette smoking doubles the risk of coronary heart disease, the number one killer of women in the United States.[2]

DETAILED DESCRIPTION

Lung cancer is the second leading cause of death among American women, and cigarette smoking causes most lung cancer deaths.[3] Tobacco smoke from cigarettes is a highly dangerous substance that contains more than 200 known poisons. Every time a smoker lights up, she is inhaling these poisons. Women smokers who die of a smoking-related disease lose on average 14 years of potential life.[4]

RISK FACTORS

Cigarette smoking poses a variety of health risks to women at every stage of their lives. Specific risks associated with smoking include:

- Childhood and adolescence:
  - Reduced rates of lung growth.
- Adulthood:
  - Decline of lung function.
  - Increased risk for infertility.
  - Premature menopause.
- Pregnancy:
  - Increased risk of preterm labor and premature delivery.
  - Increased risk of an infant with a low birth weight.
  - Increased risk for baby of Sudden Infant Death Syndrome and mental retardation.
- Postmenopause:
  - Lower bone density.
  - Increased risk for bone fracture.

SYMPTOMS & SIGNS

Potential long-term affects of smoking include:

- Chronic bronchitis.
- Emphysema.
- Lung cancer.
- Mouth and throat cancer.
- Heart disease and stroke—smoking accelerates atherosclerosis, or "hardening of the arteries".
- Bladder cancer—chemicals from tobacco are absorbed into the bloodstream and leave the body through the urine. Cancer-causing chemicals contact the bladder, increasing the risk for cancer.
- Stomach ulcer—smoking may erode the lining of the stomach. Painful ulcers can result and increase the risk for hemorrhage and the formation of a hole in the wall of the stomach.

Sources:
1. Women and Smoking: A Report of the Surgeon General, 2001.
2. National Women's Health Information Center, 2002.
3. Women and Smoking: A Report of the Surgeon General, 2001.
4. Women and Smoking: A Report of the Surgeon General, 2001.

PREVENTION & MANAGEMENT

Most smokers attempt to quit several times before they are successful. Tips for quitting smoking include:

• Set a quit date in advance.
• Tell your family and friends about your plans to quit, and ask for their support.
• Cultivate new interests that do not involve smoking.
• Talk with a health care professional about nicotine replacement and medications that improve quit rates.

The health benefits of quitting smoking begin immediately and increase as time goes on.

Bladder Cancer

Chemicals from tobacco are absorbed into the bloodstream and leave the body through the urine. These cancer-causing chemicals are always in contact with the bladder, increasing the risk for bladder cancer.

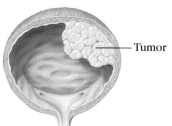

— Tumor

Affects of Smoking

Lung Cancer

Tobacco smoke is the most common cause of lung cancer. One in ten heavy smokers will get lung cancer, and in most cases it will be fatal. It is the leading cause of death by cancer because it is difficult to detect, and it is likely to spread early to the liver, brain, and bones.

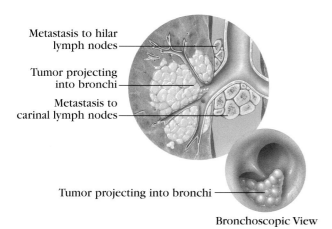

Metastasis to hilar lymph nodes

Tumor projecting into bronchi

Metastasis to carinal lymph nodes

Tumor projecting into bronchi

Bronchoscopic View

Emphysema

With emphysema, the lungs irreversibly lose their ability to take up oxygen, causing great breathing difficulty. Lung tissue loses its elasticity, air sacs tear, and stale air becomes trapped, eventually causing death from lack of oxygen.

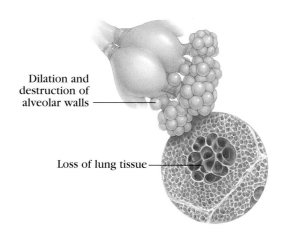

Dilation and destruction of alveolar walls

Loss of lung tissue

Fetal Risk

Carbon monoxide in smoke reduces the oxygen level in the fetus' (unborn child's) blood, while nicotine restricts the blood flow from the mother to the fetus. Smoking is thought to retard the growth of the fetus, resulting in low birth weight. Smoking also increases the risk of premature birth and infant death.

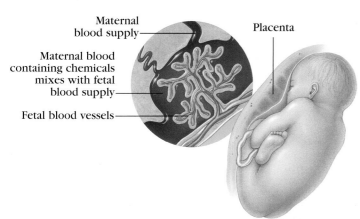

Maternal blood supply

Maternal blood containing chemicals mixes with fetal blood supply

Fetal blood vessels

Placenta

Chronic Bronchitis

A persistent cough with sputum production is the major symptom of chronic bronchitis. In the large airways, the size and number of mucus-secreting glands are increased. In the small airways, there are increased secretions, impaired handling of secretions, and inflammation that can impair or obstruct air flow.

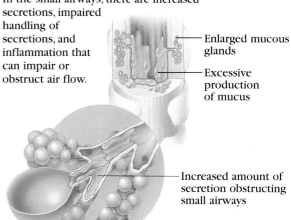

Enlarged mucous glands

Excessive production of mucus

Increased amount of secretion obstructing small airways

Glossary

Acupuncture
A procedure used in or adapted from an ancient Asian system of therapy. Its purpose is to relieve pain or produce anesthesia and involves puncturing specific body areas with long, fine needles.

Aeroallergens
Allergens (substances that cause allergies) that are present in the air.

Anaphylactic shock
A severe, often fatal form of shock typically brought on by an allergic reaction. Shock is defined as "circulatory collapse," when the arterial blood pressure is too low to maintain an adequate supply of blood to the body's tissues.

Anemia
A deficiency of the red blood cells which results in insufficient oxygen to the body's organs and tissues.

Aneurysm
A sac-like bulging of a blood vessel.

Antihistamines
Over-the-counter or prescription medications that relieve symptoms of some allergic reactions. These drugs may cause drowsiness.

Asymptomatic
Having no signs or symptoms of disease.

Atherosclerosis
Thickening of the inside walls of the coronary arteries that narrows the space through which blood can flow, decreasing and sometimes completely cutting off the supply of oxygen and nutrients to the heart.

Biofeedback
Technique that enables an individual to gain some element of voluntary control over his/her autonomic nervous system body functions. May be used to treat migraine headaches.

Bladder training
Technique that teaches people to resist the urge to urinate and gradually expand the intervals between voiding. Can involve following a timetable to store and release urine.

Breech presentation
A situation in the birthing process when the baby is not positioned head down.

Calorie
A standard unit of measurement of heat energy. Technically, 1 calorie is 1 kilocalorie, which is the amount of heat required to raise the temperature of 1 kg of water by 1 degree Celsius. The carbohydrates, fats, and proteins in food supply energy, which is measured in calories. A person's energy needs (as measured by calories) are determined by the amount of lean tissue or muscle in their body and by their level of physical activity.

Carcinoma
Cancer that begins in the skin or in tissues that line or cover internal organs.

Chemotherapy
The use of drugs to kill cancer cells.

Cholinesterase inhibitors
Drugs that inhibit cholinesterase (a chemical produced by the body that controls nerve impulse transmission) that are used in the treatment of Alzheimer's Disease to improve memory and cognitive functioning.

Colonoscopy
A procedure that allows the physician to look inside the entire large intestine, from the lowest part, the rectum, all the way up through the colon to the lower end of the small intestine.

Corticosteroids
Anti-inflammatory synthetic hormones that reduce inflammation.

Dementia
A group of symptoms caused by changes in brain function. Dementia symptoms may include asking the same questions repeatedly; becoming lost in familiar places; being unable to follow directions; getting disoriented about time, people, and places; and neglecting personal safety, hygiene, and nutrition.

Ectopic pregnancy
A potentially life-threatening form of pregnancy in which implantation of the fertilized egg occurs outside the uterus (also known as tubal pregnancy).

Electrocautery
Treatment involving the burning (cauterizing) of tissue.

Epilepsy
A group of disorders marked by problems in the normal functioning of the brain. These problems can produce seizures, unusual body movements, loss of consciousness or changes in consciousness, as well as mental problems or problems with the senses.

Estrogen
Any of several hormones that promote the development and maintenance of female sex characteristics.

Estrogen Replacement Therapy (ERT)
Estrogen-containing medications given to postmenopausal women or to women who have had their ovaries surgically removed. Hormones are given to replace the estrogen no longer produced by the ovaries. When ERT is prescribed with progesterone, the therapy is called Hormone Replacement Therapy (HRT).

Fat necrosis
Lumps of fatty material that form in response to a bruise or blow to the breast. This condition typically occurs in obese women with very large breasts.

Fibroid tumors
A benign smooth-muscle tumor, usually in the uterus or gastrointestinal tract. Also called leiomyoma.

Gestational diabetes
Gestational diabetes develops only during pregnancy. Like Type 2 diabetes, it occurs more often in African Americans, Native Americans, Hispanic Americans, and people with a family history of diabetes. Though it usually disappears after delivery, the mother is at increased risk of getting Type 2 diabetes later in life.

Hemorrhage
An escape of blood from the vessels; bleeding.

Hormonal therapy
Treatment that adds, blocks, or removes hormones. For certain conditions (such as diabetes or menopause), hormones are given to adjust low hormone levels. To slow or stop the growth of certain cancers (such as prostate and breast cancer), hormones may be given to block the body's natural hormones. Sometimes surgery is needed to remove the source of hormones.

Hormone Replacement Therapy (HRT)
Medications containing estrogen and progesterone taken to offset the symptoms and other effects of the hormone loss that accompanies menopause.

Hydrogenated fats
Fats or oils that are solidified using hydrogen; found in margarines and shortenings. Common sources of hydrogenated fats include commercially fried foods and some bakery goods.

Hysterectomy
An operation in which the uterus is removed.

IDL
Abbreviation for intermediate-density lipoprotein. IDL is one of the harmful cholesterols (like LDL) that cause heart disease. In comparison to VLDL, IDL and HDL contain a higher percentage of cholesterol.

Immunologic
Having to do with the functioning of the body's immune system (which helps fight off disease).

Immunotherapy
Treatment to stimulate or restore the ability of the immune system to fight infection and disease. It is used to lessen side effects that may be caused by some cancer treatments. In the context of treating allergies, immunotherapy is also known as allergy shots.

Intravenous
Within a vein.

Islets of Langerhans
The clumps of cells within the pancreas that include those cells that are the source of insulin and glucagon.

Kegel exercises
Exercises that can help to strengthen the muscles of the pelvis. How to do Kegel exercises: Tighten your pelvic muscles as if you are trying to hold back urine. Hold the muscles tight for a few seconds and then release them. Repeat this exercise up to ten times. Repeat the Kegel exercises up to four times each day.

Laparoscopy
A minor surgical procedure in which a laparoscope (a tube with a light in it) is inserted into a small incision in the abdomen.

Laser therapy
The use of an intensely powerful beam of light to kill cancer cells.

Lipid profile
Test that measures total cholesterol, LDL, HDL, and triglycerides.

Lumpectomy
Surgery to remove the tumor and a small amount of normal tissue around it.

Lymphatic System
The tissues and organs that produce, store and carry white blood cells that fight infection and other diseases. This system includes the bone marrow, spleen, thymus, lymph nodes, and network of thin tubes that carry lymph and white blood cells. These tubes branch, like blood vessels, into all the tissues of the body.

Macula
Also known as the macula lutea, the macula is an oval area in the retina. As you look around, light is focused onto your macula. There, millions of cells change the light into nerve signals that tell the brain what you are seeing.

Mammography/mammograms
The examination of breast tissue using x-rays.

Mastectomy—modified radical
Surgery for breast cancer in which the breast, some of the lymph nodes under the arm, the lining over the chest muscles, and sometimes part of the chest wall muscles are removed.

Mastectomy—partial
The removal of a cancer as well as some of the breast tissue around the tumor and the lining over the chest muscles below the tumor. Usually some of the lymph nodes under the arm are also taken out. Also called segmental mastectomy.

Mastectomy—total
Removal of the breast. Also called simple mastectomy.

Miscarriage
A loss of pregnancy before the middle of the second trimester.

Monoamine oxidase inhibitor (MAOI)
Type of medication to treat depression by inhibiting monoamine oxidase in the brain.

MRI
Magnetic Resonance Imaging (MRI) is a technique that uses magnets and radio waves to provide a high-resolution image of the body's internal structure.

Neurologic
Having to do with the nervous system.

Neuron
A cell of the nervous system, responsible for neurotransmission—conduction of electrochemical impulses throughout the nervous system.

Neurotransmitters
Molecules that act as chemical messengers, carrying information from one neuron to another.

Nonsteroidal anti-inflammatory drugs (NSAIDs)
A group of anti-inflammatory drugs that do not contain steroids. Used for decreasing fever, swelling, pain, and redness. Examples of NSAIDS include aspirin, ibuprofen, and naproxen.

Obstructive sleep apnea
A serious, potentially life-threatening condition that occurs during sleep, when air cannot flow into or out of the nose or mouth, although efforts to breathe continue.

Oral contraceptives
Medication designed to be taken by mouth to prevent pregnancy. Also known as birth control pills.

Ovulation
The release of an egg from an ovary during the menstrual cycle.

Palliative therapy
Treatment given to relieve symptoms caused by advanced cancer. Palliative therapy does not alter the course of a disease but can improve the quality of life.

Pancreatitis
Inflammation of the pancreas. The pancreas secretes the hormones that regulate blood sugar and the enzymes that aid digestion.

Pelvic inflammatory disease (PID)
A general term that refers to infection of the fallopian tubes (tubes that carry eggs from the ovary to the womb) and of other internal reproductive organs in women. It is a common and serious complication of some sexually transmitted diseases (STDs).

Pelvic prolapse
A state occurring when the pelvic organs—uterus, bladder, and rectum—lose their normal support and drop lower in the pelvis, often distending the pelvic floor.

Pituitary gland
A small organ—about the size of a dime and located in the center of the brain—which makes hormones that affect growth and the functions of other glands in the body.

Plant stanols and sterols
Naturally occurring compounds, found in plants, that may help reduce cholesterol.

Polycystic ovarian syndrome (PCOS)
A condition in which women may have acne, increased facial and body hair growth, excessive weight, irregular menstrual cycles, and difficulty in getting pregnant. It is thought to reflect excessive secretion of androgen from the ovaries. Androgen is a substance, usually a hormone, that stimulates the development of male sex characteristics.

Pre-eclampsia
A condition that typically starts after the 20th week of pregnancy and is related to increased blood pressure and protein in the mother's urine (as a result of kidney problems).

Progesterone
A hormone produced by the ovary. Can also be a drug, made from natural or synthetic progesterone, that can be used to control menstrual irregularities, to maintain pregnancy, and as a constituent of some oral contraceptives.

Psychotherapy
Treatment of emotional, behavioral, personality, and psychiatric disorders based primarily upon verbal or nonverbal communication and interventions with the patient, in contrast to treatments utilizing chemical and physical measures.

Pulmonary embolism
A sudden blocking of an artery in the lungs. The blockage could be caused by a blood clot or another substance, such as a fat globule, air bubble, or large piece of tissue.

Radiation therapy
The use of high-energy radiation from x-rays, gamma rays, neutrons, and other sources to kill cancer cells and shrink tumors.

RE
Abbreviation for retinol equivalents, a unit of measurement for vitamin A. 1 RE = 1 mcg. of retinol.

Renovascular
Pertaining to the blood vessels of the kidney.

Retina
The light-sensitive layer of tissue at the back of the eye that is connected by the optic nerve to the brain.

Sclerosing adenosis
A benign breast disease that involves the excessive growth of tissues in the breast's lobules.

Selective noradrenergic reuptake inhibitors (SnaRIs)
This recently developed class of drugs appears to have fewer side effects than the selective serotonin reuptake inhibitors (SSRIs).

Selective serotonin reuptake inhibitors (SSRIs)
Three of the neurotransmitters that antidepressants influence are serotonin, dopamine, and norepinephrine. SSRIs affect mainly serotonin and have been found to be effective in treating depression and anxiety without as many side effects as some older antidepressants, such as the tricyclics.

Serotonin-norepinephrine reuptake inhibitors (SNRIs)
These antidepressants affect not only serotonin (like SSRIs), but also norepinephrine, and have been found to have fewer side effects than the tricyclic antidepressants.

Stillbirth
The birth of an infant who has died prior to delivery.

Thyroid gland
A gland located beneath the voice box (larynx) that produces thyroid hormone. The thyroid helps regulate growth and metabolism.

Tricyclic antidepressants
This class of antidepressants is a predecessor of selective serotonin reuptake inhibitors (SSRIs). These medications block the reuptake (reabsorption) of the neurotransmitters norepinephrine and serotonin in the central nervous system.

Triglyceride
A form of fat in the blood that can raise the risk of heart disease.

Ulceration
The formation of an ulcer. An ulcer is a lesion through the skin or mucous membrane resulting from a loss of tissue, usually with inflammation.

VLDL
Abbreviation for very-low-density lipoprotein. VLDL carries trigylcerides and cholesterol in the blood.

On-line References (Government)

Centers for Disease Control and Prevention: www.cdc.gov

Mental Health: A Report of the Surgeon General. U.S. Department of Health and Human Services under the direction of the Substance Abuse and Mental Health Services Administration, Center for Mental Health Services, in partnership with the National Institute of Mental Health, National Institutes of Health, 2000. Available from www.surgeongeneral.gov/library/mentalhealth/home.html

NASA Women's Outreach Initiative: www.nasa.gov/women

National Cancer Institute: www.cancer.gov

National Center for Health Statistics: www.cdc.gov/nchs

National Institute of Diabetes and Digestive and Kidney Diseases: www.niddk.nih.gov

National Eye Institute: www.nei.nih.gov

National Headache Foundation: www.headaches.org

National Heart, Lung, and Blood Institute: www.nhlbi.nih.gov

National Institute of Allergy and Infectious Diseases: www.niaid.nih.gov

National Institute of Arthritis and Musculoskeletal and Skin Diseases: www.niams.nih.gov

National Institute of Mental Health: www.nimh.nih.gov

National Institute on Aging: www.nia.nih.gov

National Institute on Alcohol Abuse and Alcoholism: www.niaaa.nih.gov

National Institutes of Health Women's Health Initiative: www.nhlbi.nih.gov/whi

National Kidney and Urologic Diseases Information Clearinghouse: www.niddk.nih.gov

National Women's Health Information Center: www.4woman.org

Nutrition and Your Health: Dietary Guidelines for Americans. U.S. Departments of Health and Human Services and Agriculture, 2000. Available from www.health.gov/dietaryguidelines

Physical Activity and Health: A Report of the Surgeon General. U.S. Department of Health and Human Services, Centers for Disease Control and Prevention, National Center for Chronic Disease Prevention and Health Promotion, 1996. Available from www.cdc.gov/nccdphp/sgr/sgr.htmlSubstance Abuse and Mental Health Services Administration: www.samhsa.gov

U.S. Food and Drug Administration: www.fda.gov

U.S. National Library of Medicine: www.nlm.nih.gov

Women and Smoking: A Report of the Surgeon General. U.S. Department of Health and Human Services under the general direction of the Centers for Disease Control and Prevention, National Center for Chronic Disease Prevention and Health Promotion, Office on Smoking and Health, 2001. Available from www.cdc.gov/tobacco/sgr_forwomen.html

On-line References (Non-Government)

2002 Heart and Stroke Statistical Update. American Heart Association, 2001. Available from www.americanheart.org/presenter.jhtml?identifier=1928.

Alzheimer's Association: www.alz.org

American Academy of Allergy Asthma and Immunology: www.aaaai.org

American Dietetic Association: www.eatright.org

American Diabetes Association: www.diabetes.org

American Cancer Society: www.cancer.org

American College of Obstetricians and Gynecologists: www.acog.org

American Council for Drug Education: www.acde.org

American Council for Headache Education: www.achenet.org

American Gastroenterological Society: www.gastro.org

American Headache Society: www.aash.org

American Heart Association: www.americanheart.org

American Lung Association: www.lungusa.org

American Society for Reproductive Medicine: www.asrm.org

Arthritis Foundation: www.arthritis.org

Asthma and Allergy Foundation of America: www.aafa.org

Crohn's & Colitis Foundation of America: www.ccfa.org

Endometriosis Research Center: www.endocenter.org

Lupus Foundation of America: www.lupus.org

Mayo Foundation for Medical Education and Research: www.mayo.edu

National Alliance of Breast Cancer Organizations: www.nabco.org

National Multiple Sclerosis Society: www.nmss.org

National Uterine Fibroids Foundation: www.nuff.org

National Women's Health Resource Center: www.healthywomen.org

North American Menopause Society: www.menopause.org

Society for Women's Health Research: www.womens-health.org

Print References

Allison, Kathleen Cahill. *American Medical Association Complete Guide to Women's Health* (New York: Random House, 1996).

Carlson, Karen J., Stephanie A. Eisenstat, and Terra Ziporyn. Harvard Guide to Women's Health (Cambridge, Mass.: Harvard University Press, 1996).

Hankinson, Susan E, et al. *Healthy Women, Healthy Lives: A Guide to Preventing Disease, from the Landmark Nurses' Health Study* (New York: Simon & Schuster Source, 2001).

Miller LJ (ed). *Postpartum Mood Disorders* (Washington DC: American Psychiatric Press, 1999). www.appi.org

Stoppard, Miriam. *Women's Health Handbook: What Every Woman Needs to Know About Her Body* (New York: Dorling Kindersley, 2001).

Yates, Alison, et al. "Dietary Reference Intakes: The new basis for recommendations for calcium and related nutrients, B vitamins, and choline." Journal of the American Dietetic Association 98 (1998): 699-706.

This is just a sampling of the many Web sites that can serve as additional resources to learn more about the topics within this book.

Please note: *Information contained within this book and on these Web sites is not a substitute for professional diagnosis or treatment. Please consult with your licensed health professional to address your health concerns.*

Government Sites

National Women's Health Information Center
www.4woman.gov

National Cancer Institute
www.cancer.gov

Centers for Disease Control and Prevention
www.cdc.gov

National Institutes of Health (NIH)
www.nih.gov

Selected Institutes within the NIH

National Institute of Mental Health
www.nimh.nih.gov

National Institute on Alcohol Abuse and Alcoholism
www.niaaa.nih.gov

National Eye Institute
www.nei.nih.gov

National Institute of Diabetes and Digestive and Kidney Diseases
www.niddk.nih.gov

National Heart, Lung, and Blood Institute
www.nhlbi.nih.gov

National Institute of Arthritis and Musculoskeletal and Skin Diseases
www.niams.nih.gov

National Institute of Allergy and Infectious Disease
www.niaid.nih.gov

National Institute of Child Health and Human Development
www.nichd.nih.gov

National Institute of Neurological Disorders and Stroke
www.ninds.nih.gov

National Institute on Aging
www.nia.nih.gov

National Library of Medicine
www.nlm.nih.gov

Food and Drug Administration
www.fda.gov

Nutrition and Your Health: Dietary Guidelines for Americans
www.health.gov/dietaryguidelines

President's Council on Physical Fitness and Sports
www.fitness.gov

Non-Government Sites

Society for Women's Health Research
www.womens-health.org

National Women's Health Resource Center
www.healthywomen.org

American Cancer Society
www.cancer.org

American Diabetes Association
www.diabetes.org

American Heart Association
www.americanheart.org

American Lung Association
www.lungusa.org

American College of Obstetricians and Gynecologists
www.acog.org

American Society for Reproductive Medicine
www.asrm.org

STAFF

Liana Bauman, BA, MAMS, received her master of associated medical sciences degree from the University of Illinois at Chicago in 1998. After graduation, she worked at Biomedia Corporation as a medical-legal illustrator. Liana is now a full-time medical illustrator at the Anatomical Chart Company. She would like to dedicate her work on this book to her mother, who always encouraged her creativity.

Dana Demas, BA, contributed as a freelance writer to *Women's Health and Wellness: An Illustrated Guide*. An English major, Dana graduated from the University of Vermont and has experience in the public relations, television, and publishing industries. Inspired by many gifted female writers, she is working toward someday publishing her own creative writing. Dana would like to dedicate her work on this book to her mother, Paula, for all of her love, support, and fanatical health habits!

Dawn Gorski, BA, MAMS, received her master's in biomedical illustration from the University of Illinois at Chicago in 1998. Following graduation, she worked at Blausen Medical Communications in Houston, Texas. Missing the great city of Chicago as well as family and friends, she headed back to her hometown and is now working at the Anatomical Chart Company. Dawn would like to dedicate her work on this book to her mother, Dorothy Wieciech Gorski; her sister, Jennifer Gorski Vargo; and all of the grandmas and aunts in her family who have been an inspiration to her. They have shown her the importance of creating and sharing knowledge on women's health.

Lik Kwong, MFA, is a senior medical illustrator at the Anatomical Chart Company and currently lives in Vernon Hills, Illinois. He earned his BFA in graphic design at the University of Michigan, Ann Arbor, as well as his MFA in scientific and medical illustration. Lik would like to dedicate his work on this book to Mrs. Jean Kwong, his mother, for her love and support.

Nancy Liskar, AB, is a Phi Beta Kappa graduate of Washington University in St. Louis and a long-time resident of the Chicago area. In her twenty-plus years as a professional editor, she has enjoyed a long association with the Anatomical Chart Company and has edited consumer health publications for Women's Healthcare Consultants in Evanston, Illinois. She also has edited magazines, journals, catalogs, books, and online content for various organizations. She would like to dedicate her work on this book to her friend Lynne I., who is battling late-stage ovarian cancer with courage and humor.

Lesley Weeks Ochoa, BS, MBA, is the new product development manager for the Anatomical Chart Company. She currently lives in Chicago, but her hometown is Topsfield, Massachusetts. Lesley received a bachelor of science degree in economics from Villanova University and a master of business administration from Stanford University. Lesley would like to dedicate all her work on this book to her mother, the late Patricia Bohan Weeks, MD, as a tribute to Dr. Weeks's unflagging commitment to her family, patients, and co-workers.

Lisa Ott, BFA, is an art director at the Anatomical Chart Company. A native of Arizona, Lisa currently lives in Chicago. She earned her bachelor's in design at Columbia College Chicago. Lisa would like to dedicate her work on this book to her mother, Sylvia DeRosa, for her encouragement and support, and her aunt, Rachel Arroyo, and grandmother, the late Julia Burgos, for their inspiring strength and independence.

MEDICAL CONSULTANTS

Elisabeth A. Aron, MD, FACOG, is a Women's Reproductive Health Scholar at the University of Colorado Health Sciences Center in Denver. The Women's Reproductive Health Research program is a research training program for obstetrician-gynecologists and is sponsored by the National Institutes of Health and the University of Colorado. She earned her MD degree from the Albert Einstein College of Medicine in the Bronx, New York and completed her residency training in obstetrics and gynecology at St. Luke's/Roosevelt Medical Center in New York City. She would like to dedicate her work on this book to her daughter Andie, who inspires her to try new things every day.

William E. Burkel, PhD, is a Professor of Anatomical Sciences at the University of Michigan Medical School in Ann Arbor. A resident of Chelsea, Michigan, he received his master's and doctoral degrees at the University of North Dakota. After two years of postdoctoral work, he joined the Department of Anatomy at the University of Michigan, where he has taught human anatomy for 36 years. Dr. Burkel would like to dedicate his work on this book to his wife, Dee, whose understanding and support have made his career in anatomy possible.

Elizabeth Ann Burns, MD, MA, is a board-certified family physician and Professor of Family Medicine at the University of Illinois at Chicago College of Medicine. She currently resides in Oak Park, Illinois. She earned her MD degree at the University of Michigan Medical School in Ann Arbor and completed her family practice residency at Harrisburg (Pennsylvania) Hospital. She completed a Robert Wood Johnson Faculty Development Fellowship at the University of Iowa Department of Family Practice, and she received her MA from the university's College of Education. Dr. Burns would like to dedicate her work on this book to her mother, Genevieve Elizabeth Lombard Burns.

Cheryl Carmin, PhD, is an Associate Professor of Clinical Psychology in Psychiatry at the University of Illinois at Chicago, where she directs the Stress and Anxiety Disorders Clinic and the Cognitive Behavior Therapy Program. She completed her doctoral studies at the University of Minnesota and her postdoctoral fellowship at Case Western Reserve University Medical School and University Hospitals of Cleveland, where she specialized in the cognitive behavioral treatment of anxiety disorders. She is a Founding Fellow of the Academy of Cognitive Therapy. Dr. Carmin would like to dedicate her contribution to this book to her sister, both for her support and for her advocacy for patients' rights.

Seymour Diamond, MD, is Director of the Diamond Headache Clinic and lives in Chicago. He is a graduate of the Chicago Medical School, now located in North Chicago, Illinois. He was the first recipient of the Certificate of Added Qualification in Headache Management by the National Board for Certification in Headache Management, Moorestown, New Jersey. He would like to dedicate his work in this book to his wife, Elaine Diamond, for her continuous support.

David A. Fishman, MD, is a board-certified gynecologic oncologist and Professor of Obstetrics and Gynecology at Northwestern University in Chicago. He is the Director of the National Ovarian Cancer Early Detection Program and Director of Gynecologic Oncology Research at the Robert H. Lurie Comprehensive Cancer Center. He earned his MD at Yale University School of Medicine. Dr. Fishman would like to dedicate his work on this book to those individuals committed to improving women's health care.

Mark Hutchinson, MD, is Associate Professor of Orthopaedics and Director of Sports Medicine Service at the University of Illinois at Chicago, where he earned his MD. Dr. Hutchinson completed a fellowship in sports medicine in 1993 with Kentucky Sports Medicine and currently serves on the Board of Trustees of the American College of Sports Medicine. He would like to dedicate his work in this book to Mary Lloyd Ireland, a leader and model to many and a personal mentor who instilled in him a desire to offer elite and complete care for athletes and patients.

David A. Lipson, MD, is an Instructor in Medicine in the Pulmonary, Allergy, and Critical Care Division at the University of Pennsylvania in Philadelphia. He serves as the Director of the Obstructive Lung

Disease Program at Penn. Dr. Lipson completed his undergraduate work at the University of Pennsylvania and obtained his MD degree at Jefferson Medical College in Philadelphia. Dr. Lipson subsequently returned to Penn for his residency in medicine and pulmonary training. The American Board of Internal Medicine currently certifies him in medicine, pulmonary disease, and critical care. Dr. Lipson would like to dedicate his work on this book to his family–Beth, Sarah, and Jeffrey–without whose support his work would not be possible.

Anna L. Meenan, MD, FAAFP, is a board-certified family practitioner and Assistant Professor of Family and Community Medicine at the University of Illinois College of Medicine. A resident of Cherry Valley, Illinois, she earned her MD at the University of Illinois College of Medicine and completed her residency at the University of Illinois Rockford Medical Education Foundation in Rockford, Illinois. Dr. Meenan would like to dedicate her work on this book to her fifth-grade teacher, Miss Dougherty, who made her a scholar, and to her mother, Elna Loska, RN, BSN, who encouraged her to become a doctor.

Laura J. Miller, MD, is a board-certified psychiatrist who is Chief of Women's Services and Associate Professor of Psychiatry at the University of Illinois at Chicago. She earned her MD at Harvard Medical School and completed her residency training at the University of Chicago. Dr. Miller would like to dedicate her work on this book to her mother, Eleanor Schenk, who got her started on her quest to understand women's minds and bodies.

Ali I. Musani, MD, is an Interventional Pulmonologist at the Hospital of the University of Pennsylvania, Philadelphia. After completing a fellowship in pulmonary and critical care medicine, he received specialized training in interventional pulmonology and thoracic oncology. He would like to dedicate this work to his mother for her unconditional support and love.

Jennifer O'Rourke, RN, MSN, NP, is a board-certified family nurse practitioner at Northwestern Memorial Hospital in Chicago. She earned her NP degree at the University of Illinois at Chicago.

A resident of Chicago, Ms. O'Rourke has spent the last six years working in women's health care. She would like to acknowledge Jill Vanwormer and Ginger Rapp for the influence they have had on her career.

Bennett E. Roth, MD, is Professor of Medicine and Chief of Clinical Affairs of the Division of Digestive Disease at the UCLA School of Medicine in Los Angeles. Dr. Roth received his BS degree from Muhlenberg College in Allentown, Pennsylvania, and his MD from Hahnemann University School of Medicine in Philadelphia. He did his postgraduate training at the University of Pennsylvania and UCLA.

Michelle D. Seelig, MD, lives in Philadelphia and is a family practice resident at the University of Pennsylvania. She earned her MD at Mount Sinai School of Medicine in New York City. Dr. Seelig would like to dedicate her work on this book to Drs. Tamara Bavendam and Eileen Hoffman, her mentors and role models.

Marla C. Solomon, RD, LD, CDE, is part of a diabetes team (adult/pediatrics, obstetrics/gynecology) at Evanston Northwestern Healthcare in Skokie, Illinois. She completed her undergraduate degree in nutrition and medical dietetics at the University of Illinois at Chicago Cooperative Undergraduate Program. This included a dietetic internship at various Chicago-area hospitals. Assisting women with diabetes concerns, she has been on a diabetes team for the past eleven years. She is dedicating her work to the many women with diabetes who struggle with weight loss, as well as the women who are attempting to prevent diabetes by changing their lifestyle behaviors.

Linda Van Horn, PhD, RD, is Professor of Preventive Medicine and a Research Dietitian at Northwestern University's Feinberg School of Medicine in Chicago. She earned her undergraduate degree in dietetics from Purdue University in Indiana. Her master's degree is in exercise physiology from the University of Pittsburgh and her doctorate is in public health from the University of Illinois at Chicago. Dr. Van Horn credits her mother as the inspiration behind her initial interest in nutrition.